Effective Documentation for Occupational Therapy

Edited by Jane D. Acquaviva, OTR

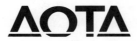

The American Occupational Therapy Association, Inc.
Rockville, Maryland

This publication is designed to provide accurate and authoritative information in regard to the subject matter covered. It is sold with the understanding that the publisher is not engaged in rendering legal, accounting, or other professional service. If legal advice or other expert assistance is required, the services of a competent professional person should be sought. *From a Declaration of Principles jointly adopted by a Committee of the American Bar Association and a Committee of Publishers.*

Printed in the United States of America

ISBN 0-910317-85-2

Director of Publications: Anne M. Rosenstein
Editor: Duncan Clark
Design: Robert Sacheli

Contents

1. If I Had Known Then What I Know Now...

Dorothy Wilson, OTR, FAOTA

The former director of a large occupational therapy department reflects on the challenges of documentation. Her frustrations are not unusual, as many managers face similar dilemmas. However, the author now has a new vantage point that makes everything clearer. As a consultant to Blue Cross of California, she reviews medical records. She never sees the patient, the therapist, or perhaps even the facility. Her knowledge of the case is only what she can glean from the medical record. Because of her work in medical review, she now understands how she could have helped her staff write more concise notes.

Dorothy J. Wilson is an occupational therapy consultant and researcher, Rancho Los Amigos Medical Center, Downey, CA.

Creating an environment that facilitates change and guiding the course of that change can be two of the most difficult management tasks. This fact was really brought home to me when I tried to change the documentation methods of a large occupational therapy department in an acute rehabilitation hospital.

The need for change became apparent during my last 4 years as director of this department. The mountains of paper continued to grow, and the documentation consumed more and more of the time that staff should have spent in direct patient care. Although hospital administration approved requests for additional staff to handle both the patient treatment and the documentation, my frustration increased. In spite of the enormous amount of time spent in documentation, the product failed to produce a coherent picture of the occupational therapy services rendered or the patient outcome. Therapists seemed compelled to document every detail so minutely that no one would read it. All the knowledge about occupational therapy services that resulted in improvement in patients' function was lost in verbiage. Computers and word processing software programs were initiated to save time with the process, but the extra time was promptly used to write more.

Although time was not saved by any process initiated, the goal that I hoped to achieve with our documentation was the ability to use the information for assistance in treating patients and as data for clinical research. Unfortunately, several peer review and audit procedures revealed that even this limited goal was not achieved.

New Insights

If a second chance to change documentation methods in this situation were to magically appear, there are several things that could be done differently. Of course, these new ideas come from the genius of hindsight.

The first step would be to develop training programs for the staff to increase their interview skills. The training would focus on how a therapist uses education, explanation, probing, and questioning during an initial interview with the patient/caregivers to identify realistic, practical, and achievable functional goals. This training would continue until the whole staff had adopted an almost religious focus on patient goals.

This is very difficult for therapists in an acute inpatient setting because most patients who are asked what they would like to achieve during their hospital stay respond with statements such as "get well" or "walk out of here." However, if we are to produce documentation that is concise and relevant, this is where the process must start. If therapists can use their professional skills to initially identify and agree on realistic outcomes that can be achieved through occupational therapy intervention, those goals would shape our documentation.

The next step in the master plan for improved documentation would be to develop and refine therapists' observation skills to their highest possible level. Following the interview, the therapists should identify underlying factors that limit functional performance by observation of the patient's attempt to perform functional tasks.

The third step in this blueprint for change would be easy. It involves expertise already demonstrated by therapists: assessment of the patient's underlying problems that limit performance. Hopefully the amount of testing and other measures used, and the resulting detail, would be cut in half by the focus developed through successful completion of the first two steps. Specific assessment of factors limiting performance should become more efficient if the functional goals and limitations are already clearly defined. The initial assessment gives us the baseline objective measures that will be used to monitor the patient's functional progress.

Initial Assessment Report

After selecting the unique occupational therapy media and procedures needed to either alleviate or compensate for the identified deficits, we are finally ready to document. The evaluation or initial assessment report would contain these three major elements: (1) mutually agreed, achievable functional goals, (2) problems amenable to occupational therapy intervention, and (3) the therapy strategy (treatment plan). These elements could be "garnished" with the length of time predicted to achieve the desired outcome and the frequency of treatment needed to reach the goals by the projected discharge date.

Subsequent progress reports would address how far we've come toward the goals and how far we still have to go. There is no need to repeat the plan of treatment unless goals are changed or new goals are identified.

The rosy glow of hindsight allows one to take advantage of every mistake made or observed during the process of attempting to change a department's documentation methods. However, I am convinced that this blueprint for change would be an effective and less frustrating way to make that change. As therapists add improved interview and observation skills to already excellent assessment and instructional skills, the process of relating functional goals, underlying factors, and the occupational therapy treatment plan in documentation should become the natural course of action. The need to report every detail of our professional process would diminish as we begin to communicate clear, relevant, and meaningful information to physicians, professional colleagues, patients, families, caregivers, third party payers, and each other.

2. Orientation to Payment

Susan Jane Scott, OTR
Frederick P. Somers

An overview of payment sources is provided because of the strong link between documentation and payment. Coverage of occupational therapy by third party payers beyond federal programs such as Medicare varies from state to state and plan to plan. This chapter provides an excellent overview, but further investigation in your own state will be necessary to have a true picture of reimbursement for your services.

Because Medicare is the largest third party payer and monitors coverage more closely than any other insurance program, other third party payers tend to follow actions made by Medicare. Therefore, it is important to understand and follow Medicare policy.

Susan Jane Scott is a legislative consultant in the legislative and political relations department of the American Occupational Therapy Association.

Frederick P. Somers is the director of the legislative and political relations department of the American Occupational Therapy Association.

Payment for occupational therapy services is derived from a variety of sources, including federal, state, private, and commercial insurers and some individuals who pay out of pocket. Funds are available through two basic kinds of payment systems: insurance programs and grant programs. Insurance programs such as Medicare, Medicaid, workers' compensation, and private plans pay providers after the service is delivered. Grant programs such as the Individuals with Disabilities Education Act (PL 94-142), the Community Mental Health Center Act, the Older Americans Act, and Social Security Title XX–Social Services Block Grant Program include occupational therapy as part of an overall program for a specified population. These two types of payment systems are vastly different. Insurance programs are highly structured, with stringent guidelines regarding which services are covered, in what settings, and by whom. Grant programs are more flexible, allowing private, state, or local entities to provide specially designed programs as long as they meet broad national goals.

All payment systems regulate the provision of services. In some cases the regulations are very strict, defining everything from the nature of the service to the average number of service units expected to be provided to a patient with a particular diagnosis. Other systems, such as health maintenance organizations (HMOs), are fairly heavily regulated regarding enrollment practices and eligibility requirements but may, for the most part, provide services in the manner they choose.

The amount of regulation is usually related directly to the cost of the care and not necessarily the quality. For example, a state Medicaid program may limit occupational therapy for a particular patient to nine visits in the home setting, deeming nine visits to be as many as are medically necessary. That arbitrary limit is imposed to keep costs down. It has little to do with the number of treatments that would benefit the patient.

In advance of treatment, occupational therapy practitioners are not liable for knowing whether a patient's health plan will cover the service. In fairness, however, therapists should be familiar with the occupational therapy coverage of various plans in the area and let their patients know up front whether their occupational therapy is covered. To do this, occupational therapists must determine as completely as possible the coverage of occupational therapy in all settings by all payers in their locality.

Federal Payment Systems

This chapter examines the various forms of payment for occupational therapy services and the guidelines and limitations that go along with them. Payment systems are divided into federal, state, and private. Government payment systems may change from time to time as Congress frequently modifies existing programs.

Medicare

Established by Congress in 1965 as Title XVIII of the Social Security Act, Medicare is by far the largest single payer for occupational therapy services. Beneficiaries of the program are the nation's elderly, 65 years of age and older; people who are disabled; and most people with end-stage renal disease. An estimated 25% of the occupational therapy profession serves Medicare beneficiaries in hospital inpatient and outpatient settings, physicians' offices, skilled nursing facilities, comprehensive outpatient rehabilitation facilities, hospices, rehabilitation agencies and clinics, and through home health agencies and private practice. The program consists of two parts: Part A–Hospital Insurance Program that pays for hospital inpatient, skilled nursing facility, home, and hospice care; and Part B–Supplementary Medical Insurance Program that covers hospital outpatient, physician, and other professional services. The coverage requirements for occupational therapy services under these two parts are discussed below.

Part A—Hospital Insurance Program
Occupational therapy services are covered under Part A when provided to eligible beneficiaries who are inpatients of hospitals and skilled nursing facilities, patients receiving posthospital home health services from a home health agency participating in Medicare, or patients receiving hospice care.

Until October 1983, Medicare paid hospitals on a retrospective basis for reasonable costs incurred in providing specific services (such as occupational therapy) to inpatients. Since that time, under the Prospective Payment System (PPS), hospitals receive a predetermined fixed sum for each discharged patient. This sum is set according to a schedule of diagnosis related groups (DRGs). Hospitals now choose which services to provide to inpatients, and occupational therapy is one of the services that may be provided. Some hospitals—psychiatric, rehabilitation, pediatric, and long-term-care—are temporarily exempt from the PPS, as are psychiatric and rehabilitation units of acute care general hospitals. These facilities and units continue to be paid retrospectively on a reasonable cost basis, and occupational therapy is a reimbursable service.

The Medicare law specifically identifies occupational therapy as a covered skilled nursing and home health service under Part A. In a home care setting, the need for intermittent skilled nursing care, physical therapy, or speech therapy alone qualifies a homebound patient for the home health benefit, but the need for occupational therapy alone does not. However, Medicare patients may continue to receive occupational therapy services under the home health benefit after their need for skilled nursing, physical therapy, or speech therapy ends.

The following limitations and qualifying conditions apply in the Part A program:

- All services must be prescribed by a physician and furnished according to a written plan of care approved by the physician.
- To qualify for skilled nursing inpatient benefits, patients must need either skilled nursing care or skilled rehabilitation services or any combination of the two on a daily basis. (The need for and provision of such

services at least 5 days a week will satisfy the "daily basis" requirement.)

- For posthospital home health services, a plan of care for the patient must be established within 14 days after the patient's discharge from a hospital or skilled nursing facility. This plan must be reviewed periodically by the physician who is responsible for the patient. A plan for occupational therapy would be a part of the overall plan.

Part A covers hospice care for eligible Medicare beneficiaries who have been certified by a physician as "terminally ill," defined in the regulations as a medical prognosis of fewer than 6 months to live. The benefit consists of three "election periods"—two of 90 days and a subsequent one of 30 days—that a beneficiary may use during his or her lifetime. A patient who elects to receive hospice benefits must waive inpatient Medicare benefits during the election period. Effective January 1, 1990, a subsequent period of coverage for hospice care beyond the 210-day limit is available if the beneficiary is recertified as terminally ill by the medical director or the physician member of the hospice program.

Medicare defines a hospice as a public agency or a private organization that is primarily engaged in providing care to terminally ill people and that meets Medicare's conditions of participation for hospices. Included are hospice centers, hospitals, special units of hospitals, skilled nursing facilities, home health agencies, and comprehensive outpatient rehabilitation facilities.

Medicare regulations for hospices mandate that four core services be available to patients 24 hours a day: counseling, nursing, physician services, and social services. The hospice is also required to provide, on an as-needed basis, occupational therapy, physical therapy, speech-language therapy, home health aids, homemaker services, and medical supplies, either directly or under a contractual arrangement.

The hospice regulations describe the purposes of occupational therapy services as controlling a patient's symptoms or enabling a patient to maintain activities of daily living and basic functional skills. All hospice employees and additional services providers, such as occupational therapists, must be licensed, certified, or registered in accordance with applicable state laws.

Hospice benefits are paid on a prospective basis. The rates, which are updated annually, are based on four primary levels of care corresponding to the degree of illness and the amount of care required.

Psychiatric occupational therapy services are covered on a hospital inpatient basis under a provision of Part A that requires hospitals to have a sufficient number of qualified therapists to provide comprehensive therapeutic activities for psychiatric inpatients. The beneficiary must have a psychiatric diagnosis, and coverage of services to an inpatient with a psychiatric diagnosis is limited to 190 days over the life of the beneficiary.

Part B—Supplementary Medical Insurance Program
Occupational therapy services are covered as Part B outpatient services when furnished by or under arrangements with any Medicare-certified provider (e.g., hospital, skilled nursing facility, home health agency, rehabilitation agency, clinic, public health agency). Outpatient occupational therapy services may be furnished by these providers to a beneficiary in the home, in the provider's outpatient facility, or to inpatients of other institutions under certain circumstances.

Part B outpatient occupational therapy services may also be furnished to beneficiaries by a Medicare-certified occupational therapist in independent practice when provided by the therapist or under the therapist's direct supervision in his or her office or in the patient's home (including a place of residence used as the patient's home, other than an institution engaged primarily in furnishing skilled health care services). Payment for outpatient occupational therapy services furnished by a Medicare-certified occupational therapist in independent practice is limited to $750 in incurred expenses annually per beneficiary. (This limit was increased from $500, effective January 1, 1990.)

Outpatient occupational therapy services are also covered under Part B of Medicare as incidental to a physician's services when rendered to beneficiaries in a physician's office or physician-directed clinic. The therapist providing the services must be employed (either full- or part-time) by the physician or the clinic, and the therapy services must be furnished under the physician's direct supervision. The physician's presence in the office or clinic satisfies the supervision requirement. Other requirements are that the therapy services be directly related to the condition for which the physician is treating the patient and that the services be included on the physician's bill to Medicare.

Outpatient occupational therapy services are also covered under Part B as comprehensive outpatient rehabilitation facility (CORF) services. A CORF is a public or private institution that is primarily engaged in providing (by or under the supervision of physicians) diagnostic, therapeutic, and restorative services on an outpatient basis for the rehabilitation of injured, sick, or disabled people. There is no requirement that occupational therapy services be furnished at any single, fixed location, so such services may be provided on-site at the CORF or off-site (i.e., the patient's home).

Occupational therapy services furnished to a beneficiary with a psychiatric diagnosis are covered under Part B of Medicare. For Medicare purposes, such a diagnosis means specific psychiatric conditions described in the *Diagnostic and Statistical Manual of Mental Disorders* (DSM-III-R)(American Psychiatric Association, 1987). Payment under Part B for all services furnished in the treatment of a patient with a psychiatric diagnoses is limited to 62.5% of the actual expenses incurred in a calendar year (prior dollar limitations in effect for Part B services furnished to psychiatric patients were repealed January 1, 1990).

Occupational therapy services furnished to a patient with a psychiatric diagnosis by a Medicare-certified occupational therapist in independent practice fall within the scope of the overall $750 annual limit per beneficiary for services rendered under this benefit.

Partial hospitalization services connected with the treatment of a beneficiary with a psychiatric diagnosis (hospital-based or affiliated psychiatric day programs) are also covered under Part B of Medicare. These services are covered only if the beneficiary would otherwise require inpatient psychiatric care. Under this benefit, Medicare covers occupational therapy services. Such services must be reasonable and necessary for the diagnosis or active treatment of the beneficiary's condition. The services must be reasonably expected to improve or maintain the beneficiary's conditions and functional level and to prevent relapse or hospitalization. The course of treatment must be prescribed, supervised, and reviewed by a physician.

Conditions for Coverage of Outpatient Occupational Therapy Services
To be reimbursable under the Medicare program, Part B outpatient occupational therapy services must meet all of the following requirements:

- The occupational therapy services must meet the conditions set forth in the Medicare coverage guidelines for such services. Included in these guidelines are requirements that the services be prescribed by a physician, be performed by a qualified occupational therapist or a qualified occupational therapy assistant under the general supervision of a qualified occupational therapist, and be reasonable and necessary for treatment of the patient's illness or injury.
- The outpatient occupational therapy services must be furnished under a written plan of treatment established either by the physician after consultation with the occupational therapist or by the therapist who will provide the services.
- A physician must certify the need for the services and that the services are or were furnished while the patient was under his or her care. There must be evidence in the clinical record that the patient has been seen by the physician at least every 30 days, and the physician must recertify at least once every 30 days that there is a continuing need for the occupational therapy services.

Medicare Conditions of Participation
To participate in the Medicare program, a provider (e.g., hospital) or supplier (e.g., occupational therapist in independent practice) of services must be certified as meeting Medicare Conditions of Participation as well as complying with all relevant state and local requirements. The Conditions of Participation are monitored and periodically revised by the Health Care Financing Administration (HCFA), the agency within the U.S. Department of Health and Human Services (HHS) that administers Medicare.

Hospitals accredited by the Joint Commission on Accreditation of Healthcare Organizations (JCAHO) or the American Osteopathic Association are deemed to have met the Conditions of Participation. Other hospitals and skilled nursing facilities, home health agencies, rehabilitation agencies, clinics, comprehensive outpatient rehabilitation facilities, and occupational therapists in independent practice are surveyed by state health agencies and certified using HCFA guidelines and Conditions of Participation specific to the type of provider or supplier.

Under modifications made in 1986 to the Medicare Conditions of Participation for hospitals, the requirement that occupational therapy practitioners meet American Occupational Therapy Association (AOTA) certification requirements was removed. The regulations now require that such personnel meet qualifications specified by a facility's medical staff that are consistent with state law. In home health agencies and comprehensive outpatient rehabilitation facilities, occupational therapy services must be provided by occupational therapists or occupational therapy assistants who are eligible for certification by AOTA. Recent changes in skilled nursing facility regulations require occupational therapy personnel to meet state regulatory requirements. In all Medicare settings, personnel must be state licensed or certified where applicable.

Medicare guidelines applicable to all settings note that while the skills of a qualified occupational therapist are required to evaluate a patient's level of function and develop a treatment plan, a qualified occupational therapy assistant may implement the plan under the general supervision of the occupational therapist. General supervision is defined by Medicare guidelines as initial direction and periodic inspection of the actual activity. The supervising occupational therapist need not always be physically present or on the premises (HCFA, 1986).

Durable Medical Equipment
Expenses incurred by a beneficiary for the rental or purchase of durable medical equipment are reimbursable if the equipment is used in the patient's home and if it is necessary and reasonable to treat an illness or an injury or to improve the functioning of a malformed body member. Medicare defines durable medical equipment as that which can withstand repeated use, is primarily and customarily used to serve a medical purpose, and generally is not useful to a person in the absence of illness or injury. An example is oxygen-assistance breathing equipment. Raised toilet seats and bathtub grab bars are not covered because they are not considered medically necessary.

Medicare Payment for Occupational Therapy Services
In 1975, HCFA (then the Bureau of Health Insurance) issued guidelines for Medicare payment of occupational therapy services. These guidelines apply to all settings in which occupational therapy is a covered service. Claims for and documentation of occupational therapy services should clearly reflect the elements of the guide-

lines, or payment may be delayed or denied. Intermediaries and carriers (insurance companies that administer Medicare claims) are bound by these guidelines, so denials that conflict with them should be strongly challenged.

The Civilian Health and Medical Program of the Uniformed Services (CHAMPUS)

CHAMPUS is a U.S. Department of Defense program of health care for the dependents of active duty members of the armed forces and for retired members. It shares the cost of medical and other health care that eligible beneficiaries receive from civilian sources. For dependents, CHAMPUS is considered the last payer, so if other coverage exists, it must be used first. The CHAMPUS program pays for services through fiscal intermediaries such as Blue Cross/Blue Shield. CHAMPUS coverage is provided under a basic program and a special program of rehabilitative benefits.

The Basic Program

Under the basic program, CHAMPUS beneficiaries can obtain both inpatient and outpatient medical and mental health care from civilian sources. Until the fall of 1984 the basic program covered occupational therapy only on a hospital inpatient basis, specifically excluding coverage in any other settings. However, federal regulations published September 14, 1984, expanded medical and mental health coverage for occupational therapy to hospital outpatient settings.

To qualify for payment, occupational therapy services must be deemed medically necessary by a supervising physician, and they must be intended to help the patient overcome or compensate for disability resulting from illness, injury, or the effects of a CHAMPUS-covered condition. The occupational therapist must be an employee of a CHAMPUS-authorized provider and must render the services in connection with CHAMPUS-authorized care in an organized inpatient or outpatient rehabilitation program. The employing institution must bill for the services (CFR, 1988, 32, §199.4).

The Special Program of Rehabilitative Benefits

The special program offers rehabilitative benefits for seriously physically handicapped and moderately or severely mentally retarded spouses and children of active duty members. Coverage is provided on an inpatient and outpatient basis, but the requirements for a beneficiary to qualify for the benefits are extremely stringent. Under this program the beneficiary pays only a small deductible. A handbook distributed by CHAMPUS provides details about coverage and payments (CHAMPUS, 1986).

Federal Employees Health Benefit Program

The Federal Employees Health Benefit Program covers federal government employees and retirees. The program is implemented by more than 350 private plans, including two that are governmentwide, several that are sponsored by employee organizations, and many that are local, comprehensive plans (such as HMOs). The federal law and regulations governing the scope of the services that must be provided do not specify particular services but only general ones, such as hospital, surgical, medical, and others. The coverage of specific services, such as occupational therapy, and the settings in which they may be provided are determined by each plan. As a general rule, the plans cover nonpsychiatric occupational therapy services in hospital inpatient settings and, to some extent and indirectly, psychiatric service. The plans vary in their coverage of occupational therapy in other settings, especially outpatient.

State Payment Systems

Medicaid

Medicaid, Title XIX of the Social Security Act, is a joint federal–state program that provides health care to the poor and the medically indigent. States have a great deal of flexibility in the definition of "medically indigent" and in the makeup and administration of the program, so benefits vary significantly from state to state. States must include all recipients of Aid to Families with Dependent Children (AFDC) and most beneficiaries of Supplementary Security Income (SSI). Not all states provide Medicaid coverage for the medically needy. Some states have a spend-down provision under which families with moderately high incomes may become eligible for Medicaid when their medical expenses reduce their income below the state standard.

Medicaid services fall into two categories: mandatory and optional. Mandatory services are ones that a state must provide to qualify for federal matching funds. Mandatory services include hospital services; laboratory work and X-rays; skilled nursing facility services; physician services; early and periodic screening, diagnosis, and treatment (EPSDT) services for those under 21; and family planning. Optional services are those that the state may choose to provide. Occupational therapy is one, along with physical therapy, speech therapy, drugs, psychiatric care, and others. The option includes psychiatric occupational therapy services. Some states have decided to cover occupational therapy services in various ways, and others have not. In 1988, Congress approved legislation to allow school systems to bill Medicaid for certain related services (including occupational therapy) provided to children in schools. In 1989, Congress broadened the scope of mandated services that states must provide to children under the EPSDT program. This change requires states to provide certain services, including occupational therapy, if they are necessary to treat a condition identified during the EPSDT screening process. Coverage of these services is required even if they are not normally covered under the state's Medicaid program. In addition, nursing home reforms adopted by Congress in 1987 require Medicaid nursing facilities to provide skilled rehabilitation services, including occupational therapy, to those of their patients who require them. Information on Medicaid coverage of occupational therapy may be obtained from a state's office of medical assistance (Medicaid).

Individuals with Disabilities Education Act

Enacted by Congress in 1975, the Education for All Handicapped Children Act (PL 94–142) required that any public school system receiving federal assistance must provide any child with disabilities a free, appropriate education in the least restrictive environment. Amended six times since 1975, the act is now known as the Individuals with Disabilities Education Act. Federal grants assist state and local education agencies in fulfilling this mandate. The law entitles children with disabilities not only to special education services, but also to related services if they are needed for the child to benefit from special education. Occupational therapy and physical therapy, among other services, are related services for children 3 to 21 years of age. Speech therapy or special education may also be related services, depending on state law. Occupational therapy services must be provided by a qualified therapist, as defined in the regulatory laws of each state or in the Code of Federal Regulations (CFR, 1988, 34, §300.12) and must be directed toward helping the child benefit from special education services. Over 18% of occupational therapists and 17% of certified occupational therapy assistants provide services to students in school settings (AOTA, 1990). About half of the occupational therapists receiving payment for services under this program are salaried employees of a school system. The remainder have contractual arrangements to serve students in one or more school systems.

For a student to receive occupational therapy, it must be included as a related service on the student's Individualized Education Program (IEP). The IEP, which is mandated by law, is developed by a team that includes the student's parent or guardian and the student, if appropriate. Occupational therapy is the legally mandated service, and this must be reflected on the IEP. Treatment approaches may be identified in a treatment plan, but the service is always identified on the IEP as occupational therapy. There is no separate occupational therapy IEP or separate occupational therapy part of an IEP. The service is clearly integrated into the one comprehensive IEP.

If school personnel or parents disagree about the provision of occupational therapy or any part of special education placement or service provision as part of an IEP, a due process hearing can be requested.

Although federal law mandates the provision of services to children with disabilities and provides some monies for states to meet the mandate, the vast majority of decisions and financial support for special education are the responsibility of state and local officials and administrators. There are also state special education laws that can expand, but not restrict, the federal mandate. Occupational therapy practitioners in school settings need to work closely with local and state education officials on issues related to funding, human resources, and regulation of services.

Workers' Compensation

Workers' compensation is a state-sponsored program supported by employer contributions and administered by insurance carriers. A beneficiary receives services identified by the workers' compensation law in his or her state. As with Medicaid, the coverage of health services, including occupational therapy, varies substantially among the states. The amounts of deductibles and copayments also vary, as do the duration and scope of services. Occupational therapy practitioners providing services to people covered by workers' compensation should investigate the coverage of occupational therapy under their particular state's law. They should also check whether services are paid for according to prevailing charge, reasonable cost, or predetermined fee. In addition, workers' compensation programs frequently have their own unique coding and billing systems that must be used when billing the program.

In several states, workers' compensation programs have established maximum allowable fees for individual modalities or procedures, using a uniform description and coding system. Sometimes the allowable fee is not comparable with a reasonable charge. If this is the case, local practitioners should work with the state workers' compensation governing board to obtain adjustments in the fee schedules (Hershman, 1984).

Private Payment Plans

Taken together, the several thousand private health insurance plans operating in the United States represent the largest source of payment for health care. No single form of private insurance prevails, and coverage requirements are not necessarily similar across the plans. But three points about them may help managers and practitioners understand their operation.

First, there are profit and nonprofit health plans. For example, Blue Cross/Blue Shield Plans are nonprofit, but Aetna and Prudential are operated for profit. Both types are private, however, and must adhere to state insurance codes, which establish coverage requirements.

Second, nearly half of all employers providing health insurance in this country now self-insure at least part of their medical benefits package. Courts have ruled that these self-funded plans are governed not by state insurance codes, but by federal standards set forth in the Employee Retirement Income Security Act (ERISA). These are very general, minimum standards and do not mention occupational therapy.

Third, the many plans of Blue Cross/Blue Shield across the country are quasi-independent. No master contract governs their coverage requirements. Thus, a Blue Cross/Blue Shield plan in one state or city may have completely different coverage requirements for occupational therapy than a plan in another state or city.

Occupational therapy practitioners should investigate how their services are covered by the private insurance plans operating in their local area. Usually one or more plans tend to dominate in an area, so this information should not be difficult to obtain. Most types of private insurance plans still pay for services on a retrospective basis. This could change in the years ahead, however, influenced by the trend toward prospective payment.

Prepaid Health Plans

Many prepaid health plans are available now, and their number is increasing. A popular type is the HMO. HMOs provide comprehensive, coordinated medical services in a limited geographic area to a group of voluntarily enrolled members. For access to these services the members pay a fixed premium at regular intervals and receive services at no or minimal extra cost.

Health maintenance organizations are of three basic types: group/staff HMOs, individual practice associations (IPAs), and network HMOs. In a group/staff HMO, care is provided in one or more locations either by a group of physicians who contract with the HMO or by physicians whom the HMO employs directly. In an IPA, the HMO contracts individually with physicians, who provide services to HMO members out of their own offices. In a network HMO, services are provided by two or more group practices with which the HMO has a contractual arrangement.

Another form of HMO is known as the social/health maintenance organization (SHMO). Designed to address the needs of the elderly as this proportion of the population increases in size, the SHMO offers health and social services to enrollees on a prepaid basis. The services provided include those covered under Medicare Parts A and B, some long-term care services, and other benefits such as eyeglasses, prescription drugs, and hearing aids. All of the services are coordinated through a single system, using a combination of public and private funding. To the extent that occupational therapy is covered under Medicare Parts A and B, it is included in services provided by the SHMO.

In all of these kinds of plans the incentive to health care organizations and practitioners is to provide only necessary health care. Occupational therapy services may be included in one or more of the plans operating in an area, but that has to be determined. If the service is not included, its addition to a plan could be negotiated.

Federal regulations governing HMOs make it fairly easy and attractive for them to enroll Medicare beneficiaries. HMOs serving Medicare beneficiaries must provide all of the benefits that the Medicare law stipulates, including occupational therapy (see the earlier section on Medicare coverage, under Federal Payment Systems). The new regulations offer an opportunity for occupational therapy practitioners to expand their services and programming through these types of organizations.

A phenomenon related to HMOs is the preferred provider organization (PPO). The PPO, which first appeared in 1980, has emerged primarily as a result of two factors: the interest of business coalitions in reducing health care costs and an oversupply of physicians or hospital beds in certain areas of the country. The PPO is not an entity but an arrangement that gives preference to certain "preferred" providers. These are providers with whom fees have been negotiated, often at discounted rates. PPOs cover the services of nonpreferred providers as well but not at particularly competitive rates, and often they give consumers further incentives to use preferred providers by offering reduced deductibles, no copayments, or special benefits. Preferred providers are usually hospitals and physicians but may also be skilled nursing facilities or home health agencies.

Self-Pay

In many cases a patient needs and receives occupational therapy but has insufficient coverage or none at all and so must pay for the services out of pocket. This can be a major problem when a patient assumes that his or her plan covers all necessary medical care. The problem occurs most often in outpatient settings because occupational therapy is frequently not covered, or the coverage is vague. These possibilities underscore the importance of occupational therapy practitioners understanding the provisions of health plans in their area and talking openly about payment with a patient before any services are rendered.

Documentation

Critical to timely payment for occupational therapy services under any system is proper documentation. Most systems require a plan of treatment that has to be approved by a physician. The plan must clearly indicate the specific occupational therapy intervention proposed for the patient. Care should be taken to show the occupational therapy services as different from other services that the patient may be receiving, such as nursing or physical therapy. Progress notes should chart specific measurable patient progress, record alterations in the treatment plan, and summarize the patient's status when treatment is discontinued. The medical record may become a legal document if placed in evidence during a court proceeding, so all entries should be strictly correct and carefully thought out. The medical record also documents that services were provided, and this could be linked directly to payment in many cases. A good rule of thumb to remember is that if it isn't written in the record, it didn't happen.

Coding of Services for Billing

A subject related to documentation is the coding of occupational therapy services for billing purposes. Various payers require different systems. For Part A inpatient hospital services the Medicare program uses the Uniform Bill #82 (UB-82, formerly HCFA 1450), which includes information about the patient's age, sex, principal diagnosis, any surgical procedures, complications or accompanying conditions, and services received. Information from the UB-82 is used by Medicare intermediaries to establish a specific DRG number (from 1 through 470) for each patient at discharge. The hospital then receives a predetermined payment rate relating to the DRG number. As of July 1985, skilled nursing facilities, home health agencies, and comprehensive outpatient rehabilitation facilities must also use this system, and an increasing number of commercial insurers and state Medicaid programs are adopting it ("Health Care," 1985).

Occupational therapists in private practice or in physician's offices have sometimes used CPT codes for billing purposes. CPT, short for *Physicians' Current Procedural Terminology* (Finkel, 1991), is a listing of descriptive terms and identifying codes for reporting medical services and procedures performed by physicians. The purpose of the terminology is to provide a uniform language that accurately designates medical, surgical, and diagnostic services and provides an effective means of reliable, nationwide communication among physicians, patients/clients, and third parties. The CPT is prepared by an editorial committee and the staff of the American Medical Association with the assistance of physicians representing all specialties of medicine. The present version, CPT-4, is the fourth edition of a work that first appeared in 1966.

The CPT-4 codes form a part of another, more widely used system, the HCFA Common Procedure Coding System (HCPCS). This was developed by HCFA to satisfy the operational needs of Medicare Part B and Medicaid fee-for-service reimbursement programs. To the CPT-4 codes, HCPCS adds additional codes and modifiers developed by other professionals and insurers to meet their reporting needs. Also included are codes developed by HCFA, state agencies, and commercial carriers to meet the claims-processing needs of Medicare and Medicaid.

The HCPCS is fast becoming a national system. Blue Cross/Blue Shield Association requires all of its participating plans to use the system, and the Health Insurance Association of America has endorsed its use by commercial insurance companies ("Health Care," 1985). State Medicaid programs are expected to adopt it in the near future.

Expanding Payment for Occupational Therapy Services

Much progress has been made in recent years in expanding payment for occupational therapy services. National efforts have been successful in broadening Medicare coverage to home health, comprehensive outpatient rehabilitation facilities, hospice programs, and HMOs. Local and state efforts have resulted in better coverage under Medicaid, the Federal Employees Health Benefit Program, and private insurance plans. In 1989, the Health Insurance Association of America reaffirmed its support for inclusion of occupational therapy in insurance plans, stating "that Occupational Therapy is a professional health care service which, when used properly, can be instrumental in reducing hospital confinement, disability, and the ultimate cost of health care" (Health Insurance Association of America, 1989, p. 5).

Further expansion of payment for occupational therapy services is a collective national, state, and local effort. Critical to success is good documentation of the medical necessity and the cost-effectiveness of occupational therapy services. The efficacy data studies that AOTA has identified support these conclusions (AOTA, 1983/4). A research study underway at AOTA seeks more evidence. Also available from AOTA is a package of material that may be used to educate potential payers about occupational therapy.

Consumer demand for occupational therapy services to be included in insurance plans available to them can be extremely helpful, as can physician and other professional support. New payment sources are developing for occupational therapy personnel, such as shopping center clinics, HMOs, and industry wellness programs. Treating patients/clients and testifying as expert witnesses in disability cases are areas of occupational therapy involvement that are growing dramatically. As the health care industry changes in response to public demand for lower health care costs, occupational therapy personnel should have many more chances to demonstrate the value and cost-effectiveness of their services.

Summary

Payment for occupational therapy services is derived from a variety of sources, including federal, state, private, and commercial insurers and some individuals who pay out of pocket. Funds are available through two basic kinds of payment systems: insurance programs (e.g., Medicare) and grant programs (e.g., the Individuals with Disabilities Education Act). The former are highly structured, the latter more flexible.

Federal payments systems include Medicare, CHAMPUS, and the Federal Employees Health Benefit Program. Medicare beneficiaries are the nation's elderly (65 years of age and older), people who are disabled, and some people with end-stage renal disease. Benefits are paid under two parts of the regulations: Part A, which provides hospital insurance, and Part B, which offers supplementary medical insurance. Under Part A, occupational therapy services are covered when provided to eligible beneficiaries who are inpatients of hospitals and skilled nursing facilities, patients/clients receiving posthospital home health services from a home health agency participating in Medicare, or patients/clients receiving hospice care.

Part B covers occupational therapy services when they are furnished by or under arrangements with any Medicare provider (e.g., hospital, skilled nursing facility, home health agency, rehabilitation agency, clinic, public health agency). The services may be provided in the home, in the provider's outpatient facility, or to inpatients of other facilities under certain circumstances.

Services under Part A or Part B must be furnished according to a written plan of care approved by a physician. Some additional conditions and limitations apply in particular settings.

Since October 1983, under the PPS, hospitals have received a predetermined fixed sum for each discharged patient/client. Some types of hospitals and some units of hospitals are temporarily exempt from this system and continue to be paid for their services on a retrospective, reasonable-cost basis.

CHAMPUS is a U.S. Department of Defense program of health care for the dependents of active duty members of the armed forces, and for retired members. For dependents, CHAMPUS is considered the last payer; if other coverage exists, it must be used first. Under the basic program, CHAMPUS beneficiaries can obtain both inpatient and outpatient medical and mental health care from civilian sources. To qualify for payment, occupational therapy services must be judged medically necessary by a supervising physician. Other conditions apply. A special program offers rehabilitative benefits for seriously physically handicapped and moderately or severely mentally retarded spouses and children of active duty members. Qualifying requirements are extremely stringent, however.

The Federal Employees Health Benefit Program, which covers federal government employees and retirees, is implemented by more than 350 private plans. Coverage of occupational therapy services is determined by each plan.

State payment systems include Medicaid, the Individuals with Disabilities Education Act, and workers' compensation. Medicaid is a joint federal–state program that provides health care to the poor and the medically indigent. Benefits vary from state to state. Occupational therapy is an optional service that states may choose to cover.

The Individuals with Disabilities Education Act entitles children with disabilities to a free appropriate education in the least restrictive environment and to the related services they need to benefit from that education. Occupational therapy is defined as a related service. For a child to receive it, it must be included in the child's IEP.

Workers' compensation is supported by employer contributions and administered by insurance carriers. A beneficiary receives services identified by the particular law in his or her state. Coverage of occupational therapy varies from state to state.

Private payment systems represent the largest source of payment for health care. No single form prevails, and coverage requirements are not uniform. Most types of private plans still pay for services on a retrospective, reasonable-cost basis, but prepaid health plans are proliferating, especially HMOs. Under these kinds of plans, based on payment of a fixed sum at regular intervals, the incentive to health care organizations and practitioners is to provide only necessary health care.

In many cases, a patient/client must pay for occupational therapy services out of pocket. This underscores the need for occupational therapy personnel to understand payment systems and to talk openly with patients/clients about their coverage.

Critical to timely payment for services is proper documentation. Care should be taken to show occupational therapy services as different from others. The goals and philosophy of the payment program should be reflected in the documentation.

Several systems exist for coding services. Various payers require different systems. Two widely used ones are UB-82 and HCFA's coding system, HCPCS.

Much progress has been made in recent years in expanding payment for occupational therapy services. Further expansion is a national, state, and local—but collective—effort. As the health care industry changes, occupational therapy personnel should have many more chances to demonstrate the value and cost-effectiveness of their services.

References   American Occupational Therapy Association, Quality Assurance Division. (1983/4). *Efficacy data briefs: Outpatient stroke therapy reduces functional deterioration*, No. 1, March 1983; *Stroke rehabilitation, including occupational therapy as part of team, shows statistically significant long-term functional gains*, No. 2, July 1983; *Research shows shorter hospitalization related to occupational therapy*, No. 3, March 1983; *Rehabilitation can be cost-effective in treatment of multiple sclerosis*, No. 4, November 1983; *Research shows day treatment, including occupational therapy, adds significantly to*

Effective Documentation for Occupational Therapy

benefits of antipsychotic drugs in care of schizophrenic patients, No. 5, October 1984. Rockville, MD: Author.

American Occupational Therapy Association. (1990). *Member data survey*. Rockville, MD: Author.

American Psychiatric Association. (1987). *Diagnostic and statistical manual of mental disorders* (3rd ed., rev.). Washington, DC: Author.

Civilian Health and Medical Program of the Uniformed Services.*CHAMPUS handbook*. (1986). Aurora, CO: Author.

Code of Federal Regulations, 32, parts 190 to 399. (1988). Washington, DC: U.S. Government Printing Office.

Code of Federal Regulations, 34, part 300. (1988). Washington, DC: U.S. Government Printing Office.

Finkel, A. J. (Ed.). (1991). *Physicians' current procedural terminology*. Chicago: American Medical Association.

Health Care Financing Administration. (1986). *Medicare part A intermediary manual, part 3: Claims process* §3101.9 . Washington, DC: U.S. Government Printing Office.

Health Care Financing Administration develops uniform coding systems. (1985). *Occupational Therapy News, 39*(4), 6.

Health Insurance Association of America. (1989, July 28). Re: Update on occupational therapy. *Insurance, Managed Care and Provider Relations Bulletin*.

Hershman, A. G. (1984). Reimbursement in private practice. *American Journal of Occupational Therapy, 38*, 299-306.

3. Why We Document

Susan C. Robertson, MS, OTR/L, FAOTA

This chapter provides an overview of all the reasons why we document. It is important to note that, although we have several target audiences when we document, we can use the same strategies to communicate with all of them.

Susan C. Robertson is an assistant professor in the occupational therapy department, Towson State University, Towson, MD.

Documentation is the general term for the communication of information about a patient or client to others. There are many people who request information about the type of service, length of treatment, modalities used, and progress on functional improvement from the service provider. Different information is needed by different people and at different times in the course of treatment. How this information is communicated is the essence of documentation formatting.

The purpose of this chapter is to explore documentation from two critical perspectives. First, the key elements of documentation are outlined. The content to be included in documentation to make it effective is discussed. Second, various approaches to presenting the key information are described. The purpose of this section of the chapter is to articulate the ways in which information may be communicated and the advantages and disadvantages of each approach.

The challenge before every occupational therapy practitioner is to select the key elements to include in the documentation and then to use an existing format or develop one that organizes those key elements into a clear, concise, and comprehensive communication about the occupational therapy outcomes. A system that works well for all kinds of treatment approaches and is easily adaptable for a given individual is worth the time it takes to develop and test a documentation procedure.

Target Audiences

What is documented is contingent on *who* needs the information. Briefly, there are several target audiences for typical occupational therapy documentation. First is the *treatment team*. Sharing evaluation results, plans for intervention, progress toward goals, and outcomes is essential to integrated care for the individual. Each member of the treatment team is interested in a different aspect of the occupational therapy program. The physician, for example, may be most interested in physical capacities being developed. On the other hand, the physical therapist may be most interested in successful approaches to achieving functional outcomes so that the occupational and physical therapy programs are complementary.

Another audience in the facility setting is the *quality assurance committee or department*. Occupational therapy practitioners are part of the service delivery mechanism of the facility that is monitored to ensure that the services provided are of high quality. Occupational therapy documentation provides information used for both retrospective and concurrent review. The record outlines the type and sequence of intervention, length of treatment, outcome, and personnel implementing the program. This information is gathered to evaluate the occupational therapy program and compare it to predetermined criteria for high quality service delivery.

Yet another audience for occupational therapy documentation is the *third party payer*. Before the onset of diagnosis related groups

(DRGs), payment for services in hospitals was determined on the basis of what services were provided to achieve predefined goals. The current system of DRGs is based on what length of stay and intervention are considered normal and customary for a given diagnosis. Although the review of inpatient occupational therapy documentation may not occur at the level of the third party payer, but rather at the level of hospital utilization review, it is still essential to the payment for services. In outpatient settings, documentation may be reviewed directly by the third party payer.

Another external body that requires good communication about the type and extent of service delivery is the *accrediting agency*. Accredited facilities must meet minimum standards for documentation in order to maintain their accreditation status. This includes not only the content and presentation of records but also the maintenance of records for a certain length of time.

Another significant audience is the *patient or client*. The emphasis on patient rights, patient advocacy, and patient autonomy have brought the medical record into the hands of the patient. Careful communication about intervention goals and progress may be integrated into the treatment process and may affect the therapeutic interaction between therapist and patient.

Increasing malpractice litigation has led to another target audience—the *legal system*. The medical record is a legal document often used in court in accident and work injury cases. In the legal system, what is not written in the medical record did not happen. It is essential to write the evaluation protocol and results, treatment goals, modalities, and functional outcomes of occupational therapy intervention.

Documentation is also used by *researchers* interested in evaluating occupational therapy service delivery. Quantitative data gleaned from the medical record may describe the types of diagnoses treated, the range of services provided, the use of types of service providers, and the relationship of modalities to outcomes. The quality of the documentation has a direct effect on the quality of the research and whether the results can be generalized.

Each of these audiences needs different information about the occupational therapy evaluation, goals, progress, and outcomes. It is important for each practitioner to identify the specific individuals and groups who may be interested in the documentation of occupational therapy services. Only then is it clear what information must be communicated and what are the key elements of the documentation.

Key Elements

It is difficult to determine which of the target audiences has the greatest influence on the design and elements of the medical record. Some would argue that the third party payer has the greatest influence because without payment for services provided there would not be an occupational therapy service at all. Others would contend that the treatment team is the most influential because the quality of care is contingent on close coordination of service delivery among related personnel. Still others would argue that the legal system is the most influential because of the high risk and costs associated with malpractice litigation.

There are numerous books and articles written about the content of the medical record. Huffman (1985) has comprehensively described the basic components and specific adaptations suitable for different treatment environments, such as ambulatory care, home care, hospice programs, and long-term-care facilities. In each practice setting, the occupational therapist must contribute information to the medical record of the patient or client treated.

Given these considerations, it is possible to identify the following essential elements of the occupational therapy record:

- patient name and patient information
- diagnosis (primary and treatment diagnoses)
- physician referral
- initial evaluation protocol and results (identify prior functional level, functional limitations, and medical conditions)
- place of service
- treatment goals (short-term and long-term, identification of problems)
- progress notes, patient's response to intervention, length of treatment, duration, levels of assistance needed
- reevaluation and results, including changes in treatment goals
- status at discharge (problem resolution, functional status)
- summary of treatment
- name of caregiver
- provider information

These are the basic components of a comprehensive documentation of occupational therapy services. It is important for each practitioner to ascertain whether these are the *only* required elements or whether additional items are necessary. There are a number of areas to check to determine whether the documentation is complete.

Some states have specific requirements; some payers have specific requirements; sometimes the facility has a particular need to include additional information for quality review. In some cases, the nature of the service dictates the information to be included in the occupational therapy record. For instance, documentation for assistive technology often needs very specific technical information. (See Chapter 12 for more information.)

The key elements of the occupational therapy documentation must be determined by each occupational therapy department and should be reviewed on a regular basis to ensure that the occupational therapy documentation format is correct.

It is critical that these key components of the medical record be consistent between service providers and among facilities. For this reason, it is important to use standard definitions "to facilitate comparison of different data bases across systems and to achieve as much uniformity as possible at the national level" (Public Health Service, 1987, p. 6). To promote consistency,

Medicare has developed uniform reporting forms that other third party payers have adopted.

Once the key elements of documentation have been identified, the next step is to design a format for recording information that conveys the key elements; communicates to the various target audiences identified; and is easily usable by the occupational therapy practitioner. This is one of the most creative aspects of documentation—designing a format that includes the necessary information; requires concise, clear, and comprehensive communication; and enables the practitioner to document efficiently and consistently.

Documentation Approaches

Documentation formats may be categorized in many ways. In this chapter, they will be distinguished by their content, authorship, and presentation style. Selecting a general approach to documentation is an essential step in deciding how to organize the information into a particular format.

Source-Oriented Medical Record

The source-oriented medical record is organized in sections according to the department providing care. All the occupational therapy evaluation, treatment, and progress information is found together in the medical record, arranged in chronological order. It is easy to locate the documentation of the physician, for example, but it is difficult to determine all the patient's problems with the source-oriented medical record.

Problem-Oriented Medical Record

The problem-oriented medical record, introduced by Lawrence Weed, MD, is organized to reflect the clinical thinking and services provided for specific patient problems. Clinical problems are followed; the efforts of various rehabilitation practitioners in relation to identified problems are noted; and the progress in remediating or minimizing the problem is documented.

The problem-oriented medical record must contain four basic components: the database, a complete list of problems, plans for each problem, and progress notes. (Weed, 1971). The database contains the results of the initial evaluation, including how the information was obtained. The data about medical history, social supports, and present illness or complaints yield a list of problems that require further evaluation or intervention. Additions and changes in the problem list are made during the course of treatment. Plans for the problems indicate strategies for how further evaluation will be conducted, how the problem will be treated, and patient education. Progress notes include subjective, objective, assessment, and plan statements commonly known as the SOAP note. The objective is to describe symptoms, report measurements and observations, interpret the data, and develop approaches to remediating or resolving the problems.

The objective, interpretative, and plan sections of the progress notes provide the physician with the opportunity to describe why a particular course of action was taken and why the usual criteria for management of a patient were not followed (Weed, 1971). All of the patient's problems can be viewed as a whole, and the relationship of allied health personnel to the total treatment plan is clearly delineated. The problem-oriented medical record requires a commitment by facility personnel to learn the technique and faithfully follow its protocol.

Integrated Medical Record

The integrated medical record is organized in strict chronological order. The information from various sources is mixed throughout the chart. This format enables the reader to define all interventions that were used with a specific phase of the illness, but it is difficult to locate and compare, for example, only the entries of the occupational therapist. This makes it difficult to compare the patient response to treatment over time. Adaptations of the integrated medical record are more commonly seen. The progress notes may take the integrated form, but reports and laboratory results may be found in source-oriented sections of the chart.

Given these three approaches to documenting patient care, there are many variations in the format for communicating information. For instance, the SOAP note from Dr. Weed's system may be used as a way to organize a progress note in the integrated medical record system. The source-oriented note is commonly presented in the narrative form, but it may also be presented in a table or grid. The next section discusses the advantages and disadvantages of various formats for documentation.

Documentation Formats

To this point, the discussion of documentation has centered on the content of the medical record. How the information is presented is another important feature of documentation. Various approaches to the format for communicating information about the patient, evaluation, treatment, and progress are presented.

Before the advent of computers, documentation was done manually--a cumbersome task at best. The literature shows that there were many approaches to organizing and communicating information for the medical record. The earliest form was the narrative. Lengthy descriptions were given of patient complaints, symptoms, function, and intervention. There were no standard protocols for drafting these narratives, and they took many different shapes. Some clearly addressed patient problems, the course of treatment, and outcome. In others, information was not well-organized or clearly descriptive of the course of treatment.

Environmental pressures such as shrinking health resources, increasing productivity standards, and tighter accreditation criteria have influenced the format for documentation. There are numerous examples of charts, grids, tables, flow sheets, and forms that point to widespread efforts in most health disciplines to streamline documentation while ensuring that the professional and legal requirements are met.

While each of these is intended to decrease documentation time and increase legibility and inclusion of necessary content in the medical record, a careful critique will reveal that some formats do not include the information needed for the various target audiences defined in the earlier part of this chapter. The key information is not included or is not presented in a way useful to third party payers, accrediting bodies, or review agencies. Critics of these formats argue that insufficient information can be included on forms that limit the ability to describe actual intervention. Proponents advocate the use of predesigned and pretested formats to facilitate a consistent, comprehensive, legible communication of the key elements of documentation.

Computers have caused another look at documentation. There are descriptions of computerized documentation strategies as well as critiques of the advantages and disadvantages of computer documentation in the recent literature (Adineh, 1987; Hathaway, 1988; McDonald & Tierney, 1988; Wolf, 1987). As with previous formats, the goal is to design a format that provides sufficient communication for targeted audiences and is clear, concise, and comprehensive. Beyond this, "a good computerized care plan system will generate assignment (flow) sheets that specify, for each caregiver, the tasks he or she is to perform in order to achieve the objectives of the plan" (Wolf, 1987, p. 39). Treatment personnel can readily scan the areas to be addressed in the normal course of intervention for a given diagnosis and design a comprehensive treatment plan. The potential for generating reports about the population served, treatment delivered, optimal staffing patterns, and supply requirements is staggering.

There are many potential risks associated with computerized approaches to documentation. There may be a reduction of emphasis in the medical record on the human element, the real-life problems experienced by the patient or client. When symptoms, functional levels, degrees of assistance needed for independence, and treatment approaches used are predefined by the computer format, it can be difficult to individualize the documentation to reflect the uniqueness of the person being treated. Treatment personnel may rely too heavily on the predefined usual course of treatment and overlook particular manifestations in the individual case. All the components of the medical record cannot be stored in the computer because of the high costs of designing and searching large files.

Computer documentation may also put a burden on the payers and reviewers of claims since standard documentation formats require that the total documentation form be filled in and printed each time a note is generated, even though only a small portion of the documentation may actually change. This can generate a large amount of paperwork and require additional reviewer time to read through the reams of material. Changes in technology alter the computerized documentation system, resulting in increased costs for staff education to use the system. As the computer is used more frequently, additional risks with computerized documentation will come to light.

Formats for documentation are always evolving. It is important for occupational therapy practitioners to update their repertoire of available approaches and routinely reevaluate the usefulness and accuracy of existing formats.

Selecting an Approach and Format

The most important step in selecting an approach to documentation and a format for use by occupational therapy staff is to determine what requirements, if any, your facility uses. Many external influences, such as the Joint Commission on the Accreditation of Healthcare Organizations (JCAHO) and the Commission on Accreditation of Rehabilitation Facilities (CARF) affect how the administration organizes documentation throughout the facility. In addition, internal influences are important. The systems for quality assurance and program evaluation have a great impact on how occupational therapy documentation should be approached. Chapter 4 details how the quality assurance system can influence documentation.

Given that certain elements of documentation are required and that particular information is needed for the target audiences, the way the information is compiled and presented is the creative part of the documentation approach. Each occupational therapy department may have a different format to meet the needs of the various groups with which it communicates.

Selecting the right approach is easy. Following the steps below will ensure success:

- Determine the needs of third party reviewers.
- Determine how the facility is accredited and what information is required by the accrediting agencies.
- Determine what procedures for quality assurance are used in the facility.
- Determine what medical records procedure are used in the facility.
- Meet with occupational therapy staff to decide on the guidelines that should be followed to clearly communicate functional goals.
- Draft a format that incorporates the information that must be communicated.
- Test the instrument and revise as needed.
- Present the instrument in draft form to the groups that would typically use the information: hospital administration, fiscal personnel, physicians, medical records department, quality assurance committee, and other team members.
- Revise the instrument as needed to meet the requirements of these groups.
- Set a time period of 6-8 months to use the instrument. Plan a formal meeting to discuss the instrument, its usefulness, and ability to communicate. Make revisions as needed.
- Keep the instrument fresh by regularly checking to see if the information you want to communicate is being understood by the target audiences you have identified.
- Keep current on trends in documentation and payment for health services and adapt the instrument as needed to meet external changes.

Remembering that *form follows function* will help in keeping the paperwork down, designing a useful and usable format, and streamlining the kinds of information that need to be communicated. Monitoring the documentation process may seem to be cumbersome, but doing a thorough job on this aspect of documentation will mean less time overall in documenting practice. The ultimate goal is the provision of high quality care. Documentation is essential to meeting that goal.

References

Adineh, M. (1987). Monitoring chart completion using SPIRES. *Topics in Health Record Management, 7*(4), 68-73.

Hathaway, G.E. (1988, April). Computerized documentation strengthens risk management. *Provider*, p. 45.

Huffman, E.K. (1985). *Medical record management*. Berwyn, IL: Physician's Record Company.

McDonald, C.J., & Tierney, W.M. (1988). Computer-stored medical records: Their future role in medical practice. *Journal of the American Medical Association, 259*, 3433-3440.

Public Health Service. (1987). *Statistical aspects of physician payment systems*. (DHHS Publication No. PHS 87-1461). Hyattsville, MD: National Center for Health Statistics.

Weed, L.L. (1971). Quality control and the medical record. *Archives of Internal Medicine, 127*, 101-105.

Wolf, S.C. (1987, June). Administration: Computerized care plans a strong management tool. *Provider*, pp. 39-40.

Additional Resources

Acquaviva, J.A., & Steich, T.J. (1988). Occupational therapy documentation in mental health. In S.C. Robertson (Ed.), *Mental health FOCUS: Skills for assessment and treatment*. (pp. 1-169–1-177). Rockville, MD: American Occupational Therapy Association.

Allen, A.M. (1987). Interrogatories: Charting—the dreaded dilemma. *Orthopaedic Nursing, 6*(5), 47.

American Occupational Therapy Association. (1980). *Sample forms for occupational therapy*. Rockville, MD: Author.

Bair, J., & Gwin, C. (1985). *A productivity systems guide for occupational therapy*. Rockville, MD: American Occupational Therapy Association.

Bjorn, J.C. (1970). *The problem-oriented private practice of medicine: A system for comprehensive health care*. Chicago: McGraw-Hill Publications.

Breines, E. (1983). *Functional assessment scale*. Lebanon, NJ: Geri-Rehab.

Catton, P. (1986, October). Patient confidentiality: Peeking inside Pandora's box. *Medical World News*, pp. 62-77.

Cembrowski, G.S. (1986). Use of patient data for quality control. *Clinics in Laboratory Medicine, 6*, 715-733.

Foster, S.D. (1986). Focus on patient teaching: An innovative documentation tool. *MCN: The American Journal of Maternal Child Nursing, 11*, 419.

Gabriele, E.R. (1973). Medical record system: Acquisition and handling of clinical information. In *Quality assurance of medical care*. Washington, DC: Regional Medical Programs Service, Health Services and Mental Health Administration, U.S. Department of Health, Education, and Welfare.

Gondringer, N.S. (1986). Medical malpractice: The need for documentation/communication. *Journal of the American Association of Nurse Anesthetists, 54*, 490-495.

Grimaldi, P.L., & Micheletti, J.A. (1985). *Prospective payment: The definitive guide to reimbursement*. Chicago: Pluribus Press.

Grimaldi, P.L., & Shlala, T.J. (1986, April). Case-mix adjustments require tighter documentation. *Health Progress*, pp. 30-35.

Gropper, E.I. (1988, March-April). Does your charting reflect your worth? *Geriatric Nursing*, pp. 99-101.

Haller, K.B. (1987). Keys to research: Systematic documentation of practice. *MCN: The American Journal of Maternal Child Nursing, 12*, 152.

Hawkins, D.E. (1975). *Life skills for the developmentally disabled: An approach to accountability in deinstitutionalization*. Washington, DC: Division of Rehabilitation Medicine, Department of Medicine, George Washington University.

Minnesota Occupational Therapy Association. (1978). *Description of occupational therapy services*. Minneapolis, MN: Author.

Moriarty, Z. (1987, May). Nursing: Will your charting methods protect you from lawsuits? *Provider*, pp. 52, 54.

Morrissey-Ross, M. (1988). Documentation: If you haven't written it, you haven't done it. *Nursing Clinics of North America, 23*, 363-371.

Rabinow, J. (1988). Occupational health records: Documentation and confidentiality. *American Association of Occupational Health Nurses Journal, 36*, 314-317.

Rhodes, A.M. (1986). Focus on legal issues: Principles of documentation. *MCN: The American Journal of Maternal Child Nursing, 11*, 381.

Robertson, S.C. (1977). *The development and use of a documentation tool incorporating the occupational therapy outcome criterion in a psychiatric day treatment center*. Unpublished master's thesis, San Jose State University, San Jose, CA.

Schneider, D. (1979). *A reason for visit classifications for ambulatory care*. (Publication No. PHS 79-1352). Washington, DC: U.S. Department of Health Education, and Welfare.

Weed, L.L. (1968). Medical records that guide and teach. *The New England Journal of Medicine, 278,* 593-600.

Weed, L.L. (1968). Medical records that guide and teach (concluded). *The New England Journal of Medicine, 278,* 652-658.

Werbell, B., & Hammer, S. (1986). The bottom line: Better business decisions today for tomorrow. *Healthcare Computing and Communications, 3*(9), 74.

4. Documentation for Quality Assurance

Barbara E. Joe, MA

This chapter emphasizes the importance of documentation as a means of program evaluation or quality improvement. Documenting patient outcomes in functional terms is critical for collecting data for quality assurance purposes.

Barbara E. Joe is senior staff writer for the AOTA publication, *OT Week*.

Most occupational therapists say candidly that they chose their profession because they enjoy direct contact with people and the satisfaction that comes from helping patients improve their functioning and quality of life. Recording what takes place between therapist and patient in the medical record is considered secondary, a paperwork chore most occupational therapists fulfill conscientiously, though not always with overwhelming enthusiasm. These somewhat reluctant documenters need to become aware that documentation is not just an add-on or the manifestation of a bureaucratic whim, but a necessary element in the substantiation of treatment.

It is no longer sufficient, if indeed it ever was, for the medical practitioner to give reassurances of quality care or good treatment from an exalted or paternalistic position of authority. Health care professionals used to be able to say, "Trust me;" now patients and providers are demanding "Show us." There are external demands from all sides—from insurance companies to government to patients themselves—asking for concrete evidence that the treatment given was both necessary and proper. Quality assurance (QA) is a system designed to demonstrate quality care, and good documentation is an essential component.

The medical record, once a fairly modest sheet of paper covered with sometimes illegible scribbling, has grown in stature and sophistication to become the ultimate repository of data spun off for a wide variety of purposes. And because these data have proved so useful, new data requirements are continually being added. On the other hand, streamlined reporting formats, clerical assistance, and computerization offer prospects of lightening the documentation burden.

QA Documentation: Let Us Count the Ways

Documentation in its broadest sense is anything put down in writing or recorded in any other way, such as photo file, video, or audio tape. When a traveler keeps a diary and takes pictures, that is a form of documentation. Thus, the traditional medical record is only one possible form of health care documentation, though doubtless the most important and universal.

For quality assurance, which is concerned with patterns of care for all patients—though often examined according to separate diagnostic categories—the medical record is not the only data source. Patient satisfaction questionnaires, direct observation, incident reports, and complaints from patients or their families are examples of other sources.

Nevertheless, since this book is primarily concerned with the written documentation contained in the medical record, and since that record is the most comprehensive and universal locus of health care documentation, the focus of this chapter is necessarily on the medical record and how it can best be used for quality assurance purposes.

Quality Assurance and Documentation

The purpose of quality assurance, sometimes called quality assessment or, more recently, quality improvement, is to judge the quality of health care. Program evaluation has the same purpose. Indeed, there has been a growing convergence between "quality assurance," the name for the evaluation system used by the Joint Commission for the Accreditation of Healthcare Organizations (JCAHO), and "program evaluation," the system favored by the Commission for Accreditation of Rehabilitation Facilities (CARF). The two terms can now be used almost interchangeably.

JCAHO currently follows a 10-step quality assurance process, which can only be briefly outlined here, consisting of the following:

1. assigning responsibility
2. delineating the scope of care
3. identifying important aspects of care
4. establishing indicators of quality
5. setting thresholds for evaluation
6. collecting and organizing data
7. evaluating care
8. taking problem-solving actions
9. assessing the effectiveness of these actions through evidence of improvement
10. communicating relevant information through appropriate channels

Of these steps, documentation is especially crucial to steps 6 and 9.

Good documentation is structured to yield good information for quality assurance (or program evaluation), as well as other purposes such as reimbursement or research. There is no need for separate quality assurance documentation. However, just as there may need to be secondary or supporting documentation, apart from the primary medical record, required for treatment and payment purposes, so there usually will be separate worksheets or summary sheets for quality assurance information extrapolated from primary records.

Medical record documentation is intended to reflect treatment accurately. While treatment is not static but ongoing, documentation itself is usually not strictly continuous. Rather, it is done at regular intervals that, taken together, represent the actual flow of care in the same way that successive still frames form a motion picture. This periodic aspect of documentation applies to quality assurance as well.

Data gathering for quality assurance is often imagined to be a mysterious and highly technical process. It is not. It usually involves looking at key items in the medical record, compiling the information on those items for an identified group of patients at specified time intervals, and periodically analyzing the results. Changes, particularly those indicating a negative trend, such as a steady drop in the percentage of stroke patients able to dress themselves after a given number of treatment sessions, or increasing readmissions for mental health patients, often signal a decrease in the quality of care. At the very least, such changes must be examined, explained, and—if actual deficiencies are found—remedied.

After appropriate remedial action is taken, the process of extracting, collating, and examining the same medical record information as before and comparing the results is needed to show whether the remedy has actually had the desired improvement effect. The process of compiling this information need not be complicated and can usually be combined with other types of data gathering.

Continuous Monitoring

Because quality assurance data are needed on a regular basis, as well as before and after remedial action is undertaken, accrediting bodies commonly refer to requirements for "continuous" or "concurrent" quality assurance and program evaluation monitoring. This monitoring is nothing more than the regular documentation, measurement, and reporting of key indicators to ascertain the quality of care. The requirement for "continuous" documentation and monitoring is sometimes misunderstood, because it actually refers to notations entered according to a preestablished schedule, whether daily, weekly, monthly, quarterly, or at key junctures such as initial assessment, formulation of the plan of care, goal-setting, reassessment, discharge, and follow-up. These periodic documentation entries reflect and report on the continuous process of actual care.

Not only is documentation—whether for QA or other purposes—not strictly continuous, but it also cannot record everything. Documentation reveals a slice of life, a quick snapshot, but cannot be a detailed recreation of the complete reality. The most important, relevant items of information must be sifted out from the boundless ocean of activity and put down on paper (or into the computer). Selecting this information requires judgment. The fact that a patient's daughter visits wearing a yellow and red polka-dot dress may warrant mention only if the bright colors have made a previously listless patient sit up and take notice. This type of information, in turn, specifically becomes QA information when it is judged to be of particular importance and becomes available for a number of patients. High importance and high volume are two markers identifying health care activities as appropriate for quality assurance monitoring.

From the selected data on each individual patient actually recorded in each medical record, quality assurance becomes more selective still, concentrating on only a few key items of special importance, perhaps 5 or 10 for each identified patient group. The data in the medical record particularly appropriate for quality assurance are, as already indicated, those that apply to a number of patients, however categorized—whether by age, race, sex, diagnosis, severity of illness, treatment setting, duration of treatment, cost of care, or any other factors, alone or in combination. Large groups of patients or high-volume activities are favored for quality assurance monitoring. However, very important information for small groups of high-risk patients—for example, those with postsurgical hip dislocations—is also appropriate for QA.

The entire occupational therapy department or interdisciplinary treatment team should be involved with the initial selection of which indicators to monitor and in choosing which supporting data to look at in the medical record in relation to those indicators.

Outcomes of Care

The purpose of all health care is to produce better, more desirable results than would have occurred without any intervention. What these desirable results are is a matter of values, usually a combination of individual patient values, professional values, and social values. Independence, for example, is a core value for most Americans, but may be less accepted elsewhere, as American therapists working in the third world have sometimes discovered. Yet an almost universal goal of our own health system is to help patients achieve maximum self-direction and the ability to function with minimum assistance.

What do we see if a patient is independent? Perhaps a patient who performs ADL tasks unaided. Perhaps a patient who can live at home alone or with minimal guidance and help from another household member. Perhaps a patient who is working in competitive employment. These abilities of the patient can be verified by direct observation, testing, and reporting by the patient, family, or employer. When demonstration of these abilities is recorded in a number of medical records corresponding to a number of patients and the data are aggregated, we call it quality assurance.

The main difference between individual patient assessment and "quality" assessment is that the latter is based on all or a specified subcategory of patient records, not just one. Adverse results for a given patient may simply reflect personal idiosyncrasies or accidental factors, while consistently unfavorable results across a group of patients tend to indicate substandard care. Likewise, consistently favorable outcomes are more likely to reflect good care than does a single episode.

Insofar as treatment can be shown to have contributed to patients' abilities to function independently, these abilities become "outcomes" of care, i.e., results attributable—at least in part—to the care provided. The thrust of quality assurance activities is to demonstrate that favorable outcomes have actually occurred and to find ways to further improve those favorable outcomes, either in terms of the numbers and percentage of patients involved and/or their average progress.

Thus, continuing with the example of independence, let us assume that a combination of experience, expert opinion, and the professional literature shows that 60% of stroke patients can be expected to be discharged to their homes if provided with specified rehabilitation services—including occupational therapy of a particular intensity and duration. Without such services, let us say, only 30% can be expected to be able to go home. The 60% figure therefore indicates a result that is an outcome of care, not just something that would have happened anyway.

This figure also becomes the minimum standard of performance. If, in clinic X, only 40% of stroke patients are able to go home, then—unless there is definite evidence that patients there are sicker, older, or otherwise different from the average stroke patient—it can be concluded that optimum care is not being provided. If, however, a whopping 80% of the stroke patients at clinic X can go home, either the care is superior or the patients there are less severely affected by their illness.

For this result or any other "outcome" to be known and measured for quality assurance purposes, it must first be recorded. Each patient's discharge destination must be noted in the medical record or elsewhere. It is a necessary precondition for any outcome measurement to have relevant items individually documented to begin with. And this documentation must be accurate and credible.

Another possible way to define and measure favorable outcomes would be in terms of a reduction in the hours of activities of daily living (ADL) assistance needed by discharged stroke patients. Thus an outpatient or home health occupational therapy program might measure its success—again documented in the record—by a minimum or specified average reduction in the number of hours per week of personal assistance required by stroke patients living in their own homes. Whatever the particular outcomes documented, they must be measurable and understandable. And definitions must be consistent. Good documentation incorporates all these qualities.

Process versus Outcomes

While quality assurance documentation focuses on outcomes, it must be acknowledged that "outcomes" are somewhat arbitrary endpoints, since means and ends are not strictly separable. Thus, for quality assurance purposes, both process and outcome measurements are required. "Process" measures would apply to activities such as performing initial evaluations on all or an acceptable percentage of patients referred to occupational therapy, completing evaluations within a specified time period, developing a treatment plan for all patients, and providing a minimum number of hours of treatment per patient per day or week.

But unless such process measures are combined with measures of "outcomes," of what actually happens to patients in terms of their well-being and performance, they are not good measures of quality. Quality assurance must always go the further step of looking at what happens to patients, thus combining both process and outcome measures. It is not enough to set goals for patients. There must also be verification that these goals, or a reasonable proportion of them, are actually achieved.

What Documentation Means to QA

Good documentation yields good information for quality assurance as well as for other purposes, making separate quality assurance documentation unnecessary. However, as indicated, supplementary worksheets or summary sheets may be needed for quality assurance information taken from primary records.

Except for these worksheets or where a special study on a particular problem is required, documentation for quality assurance is not different from ordinary documentation. Most of the data needed for quality assurance can be taken from the medical record, assuming the record contains adequate information on process and outcomes to begin with.

Most of the key elements of documentation covered in Chapter 3 are essential for quality assurance. For ease of reference, they are listed again here. The first item, the patient's name, is not required for QA (QA information is anonymous and privileged), but some sort of patient identifier, such as a number, as well as information on personal characteristics (age, sex, race), is needed. The second item, the diagnosis, is clearly central to quality assurance. If there has been a physician referral, component 3, the time and date are important. Initial evaluation, number 4, is also key.

The next item listed, place of service, is not important for QA purposes, except perhaps in a generic sense, such as acute care hospital versus outpatient clinic. Treatment goals, progress notes, reevaluation results, and discharge status—the series of components that follow—are at the heart of quality assurance. These progressive measurements establish the record of individual patient progress. They record—and substantiate—quality of care. The final three items listed—summary of treatment, name of caregiver, and provider information—are usually not necessary for quality assurance. Documentation for quality assurance *does* require that proper dates and times be recorded, since prompt and timely responses to referrals and providing the best possible care in the shortest possible time are measures of quality.

Good documentation automatically reflects the quality of care, whether for one patient or many. Good documentation *communicates* relevant information in a logical sequence; it *educates* therapists by giving regular feedback concerning patients' responses to treatment; and it *provides accountability* by recording information in measurable, concise, consistent, and fairly objective terms.

There is no single blueprint for quality assurance documentation in occupational therapy or any other field. Treatment is an ever-changing process; expectations of continuous improvement are built into health care; and accrediting bodies are constantly revising their standards. Therefore, a fixed and static documentation system—"one size fits all"—is neither necessary nor desirable.

What is necessary is that principles of good documentation be conscientiously observed. These principles, as related to quality assurance, are to accurately record all important data; to provide this information in simple, consistently defined, measurable terms; and to make it easy to retrieve and collate. This is a challenging, but not impossible, task requiring careful thought, analysis, and perhaps some trial runs. However, these basic principles of good quality assurance rest ultimately on good documentation, which merely follows the same principles.

Future Developments

While there is no universal documentation system applicable to all situations, at least one quality assurance-related caveat is in order for the not-too-distant future. JCAHO has announced plans to require the continuous monitoring and reporting of certain key indicators of quality care by all health care disciplines. These indicators will be somewhat different for each profession, but the same within each.

The plan is to have fairly specific data on these indicators collected on a national basis and then to provide periodic feedback to each facility on how its own performance compares with the national average. The details and time frame for implementation of such requirements have been undergoing a good deal of revision lately. However, the field-testing of data for certain high-volume quality care indicators is now being conducted by JCAHO. Although this field testing does not yet involve occupational therapy, it is likely that a few key national indicators, requiring consistent, ongoing documentation and measurement, will eventually be mandated for occupational therapy as well as for other disciplines. This will require standardization in documentation, data collection, and reporting on these items.

When this happens, if occupational therapy departments already have their house in order in terms of documentation, the incorporation of these new national indicator monitoring requirements will be facilitated. Furthermore, those departments demonstrating good occupational therapy documentation could well end up being chosen as prototypes for the development, measurement, and reporting of these national indicators, while also providing an experience base for setting preliminary quality standards for the profession as a whole.

Another anticipated development related to quality assurance documentation concerns confidentiality. While quality assurance reports and secondary worksheets are currently privileged, this policy is coming under increasing legal challenge. It seems likely that in the future, at least some quality assurance data will have to be made public. Furthermore, the ties between quality assurance and reimbursement are apt to become more explicit over time. Thus quality assurance requirements are moving toward greater rigor, specificity, and importance in the health care system, and reimbursement is likely to become increasingly dependent on them.

Finally, JCAHO has announced plans to connect the present quality assurance system into one based on achieving continuous quality improvement (CQI), a concept also taking hold in industry. While the specifics have not been worked out, good documentation will still play a crucial role in this new system.

Poor documentation doesn't always mean poor care, but only good documentation can demonstrate good care. And demonstrating good care is finally what quality assurance is all about!

For further information on quality assurance, a good source is the AOTA publication *Quality Assurance in Occupational Therapy*.

5. Clinical Reasoning for Documentation

Claudia Allen, MA, OTR, FAOTA

This chapter looks at the thinking process behind documentation. Accurate documentation and patient/client intervention are contingent on a step-by-step process. The process must provide information that is useful for note writing as well as treatment planning.

Claudia Allen is chief of occupational therapy, Los Angeles County/University of Southern California Medical Center, Los Angeles, CA.

ocumentation is a way of communicating the value of occupational therapy services. The people who read these notes usually refer patients for services or pay for the services provided. To stay in business, therapists must be able to explain the utility, importance, and consequences of the services provided, and that requires a clear understanding of what is expected. The value of occupational therapy services is maximizing a disabled person's remaining ability to function. The ability to function is seen while a person is doing an activity. The activity must be meaningful to the individual, given his or her station in life. Occupational therapists are expected to improve the performance of activities that are meaningful to disabled individuals who have experienced a recent loss in their ability to function.

The Clinical Reasoning Process

Keeping track of improvements in activity performance is complicated because the number of underlying factors that can reduce performance is enormous. Sorting through the factors, correcting limitations that can be changed, avoiding limitations that cannot be changed, finding remaining abilities, and negotiating and prioritizing activities with patients and caregivers is a complex process. This chapter suggests a clinical reasoning process designed to help therapists keep the focus of treatment on the performance of activities that are meaningful to disabled individuals. That clinical reasoning process is outlined in Figure 5.1, which follows the text in this chapter. The 8 steps outlined in Figure 5.1 will be referred to extensively throughout the chapter.

Holding therapists accountable for producing an improvement in the quality of activity performance is a relatively recent expectation. While it is true that therapists have always claimed that the value of occupational therapy services was an improved ability to function, the actual outcome of the services provided has been ambiguous. Holding ourselves accountable for specific treatment outcomes is an emerging process with signs of improvement over the years.

Before Medicare came into effect, I remember writing treatment goals and progress notes that were seldom, if ever, read by anyone else. The positive side of that situation was that therapists learned to use documentation to self-monitor treatment effectiveness. The trouble was that it was hard to take oneself seriously if no one else seemed to care about what one was doing.

The first efforts to hold health care professionals accountable were directed toward writing measurable treatment objectives. Measurable treatment objectives had a disastrous effect on the practice of occupational therapy. It is very hard to measure functional activities and much easier to measure neuromuscular impairments like strength and range of motion. Documentation requirements made it difficult to address the individual who was experiencing the limitation. Practice became deficit-driven. One found a problem, measured it, rehearsed improvements, and measured the improvements. By focusing on measurable problems, therapists had trouble explaining the functional meaning of the problems.

During the last 2 decades the insurance industry has been encouraging therapists to be more specific by suggesting that treatment goals should be reasonable, necessary, and achievable in a predictable amount of time. While these terms are an improvement, sufficient ambiguity remains to make it hard to address functional activities. Therapists are still stuck with reducing measurable problems.

The Medicare Part B guidelines (see Book Appendices) are an effort to put the functional meaning of an activity back into practice. Therapists are asked to follow a pretest/posttest design to document an improvement in activity performance. The functional meaning of a specified activity to the individual patient must be addressed. The guidelines provide a great opportunity to get occupational therapy back on the target of functional activities if we can figure out how to write reasonable and necessary treatment goals that can be achieved in a predictable amount of time.

This chapter is designed to help therapists reorient the way they think about treatment goals. Most of the steps are familiar to experienced therapists. Emphasis is placed on those aspects that are most apt to require change in the way therapists think and provide services. The recommendations are for relearning, which is much harder than new learning. So, be patient with yourself; all of us are struggling to make this shift.

Therapists have been expected to reduce patients' problems. Now they are expected to help patients improve the performance of activities that are meaningful to the patients. The change in semantics aims at improving the outcome of occupational therapy. An analysis of the current clinical reasoning process suggests that the improvements can be made by adding 2 steps to the current process (see Figure 5.1). Current practice has been divided into 6 steps: steps 1, 4, 5, 6, 7, 8. The additions are described in steps 2 and 3. This clinical reasoning is intended for all specialty areas of practice.

Step 1   The first step is a prediction of functional outcome based on groups of people with similar problems. The medical diagnosis and the onset set a range for expected change in functional ability. Additional medical diagnoses that could restrict the range or rate of change are noted. The patient's functional history and response to previous occupational therapy treatment can also be used to establish a general prediction of the expected quality of activity performance. From this information an estimate of the discharge placement and the need for assistance can be made. What should be noted here is that predictions of functional outcomes can be made without any consideration of the individual patient, his or her culture, or the social situation. Functional outcomes are largely determined by the pathology and what nature and medicine can do to correct the pathology.

Step 2   The individual patient, his or her culture, and the social situation are factored in step 2. Occupational therapists start with an expected loss in function and begin to explore what that means to the individual. The activities that the person has done in the past, referred to as a functional history or occupational history, are identified. The therapist is looking for safety hazards that are apt to result from the functional losses that the patient and caregiver may not have considered. Activities that can still be done safely also need to be identified.

The meaning of a loss to individuals, given their stations in life, becomes apparent during the interview. The therapist must also begin an educational process about what occupational therapy services can realistically achieve. Many patients and/or caregivers have unrealistic goals in mind. Losses are hard to accept. Step 2 should begin the process of accepting losses that cannot be restored.

Step 2 is a collaborative process. The patient and the caregiver will tell you what the patient used to do before the onset of the diagnosis. The therapist can tell the patient and the caregiver how the loss is apt to affect functional activities (Allen & Earhart, 1992). Together you can begin to sketch out activities that are both achievable and meaningful.

When an impairment is recent, a denial of the disability is a frequent problem for both the patient and caregiver. A focus on short-term goals is a way of obtaining cooperation during the initial interview, but if this tactic is used, further discussion of long-term goals at a future date is advised. Therapists are often involved in the sad situation of helping people grieve over the loss of former abilities with reduced promises for the future. A neglect of the grief process tends to produce meaningless treatment goals and a sense that occupational therapy services were of no value. Step 2 is painful, but the alternative has been the provision of useless services.

Long-term goals are set within the context of loss of physical abilities, cognitive abilities, the natural course of the disease, and the available social and physical support systems. The long-term goal is an estimate of the patient's rehabilitation potential to do the activities identified in step 2. The activities selected must be acceptable to the patient and/or the caregiver.

Step 3   Step 3 is an observation of the performance of one of the activities requested in step 2. The therapist should observe performance of the requested activity and begin to think about underlying impairments that could explain the patient's difficulties. The purpose of this observation is to select evaluation instruments. Selecting evaluation instruments is a big change for many therapists who currently go through the same long lists of evaluations for all patients. Lengthy evaluations are expensive and often unnecessary. Therapists should have a rationale for the evaluation administered to each patient. The rationale should explore a hypothesized difficulty that is related to the requested activity. The time saved on unnecessary evaluations could make up for the time spent on steps 2 and 3.

Before leaving step 3 the therapist should verify the long-term goal with the patient and/or the caregiver. The therapist's estimate of the quality of activity performance should be clearly stated. In many instances the estimate of the quality of activity performance may be unacceptable, and a renegotiation of the requested activity may be indicated. In current practice, the realities of limited functional outcomes are often avoided until the end of treatment. Avoidance of unpleasant realities does not promote adjustment. Avoidance does protect the therapist from confronting reality, but this self-serving practice cannot be justified. Even with the therapist's best efforts to explain a limited potential, some people are not ready to hear bad news. We cannot make people listen, but we do have an obligation to provide the information.

Step 3 may be done with acute medical conditions where some degree of residual loss is ambiguous. The natural course of the disease and the usual response to available medical treatment are predictors of functional outcomes. Recent onset with brain impairments are probably the hardest to predict, and projections of what can be achieved within the next month or two are the most reliable. The fact that most functional change occurs within the first 6 months (after brain injury) should be explained.

Step 4   Step 4 establishes the sequence for meeting short-term goals. Changes that involve neuromuscular impairments tend to follow a similar pattern of reducing pain; preventing accidents, injuries, or complications; making neuromuscular changes; and teaching compensations for residual physical disabilities. The sequence of short-term goals for brain impairments probably follows the natural course of recovery from brain injury. Whether short-term goals are following or leading the natural course of recovery is a matter of theoretical debate within occupational therapy that cannot be resolved here (Allen & Earhart, 1992).

The issue that does need to be addressed is whether the patient can be expected to improve or not, because that affects payment for occupational therapy services. Payers such as Medicare will pay for two types of treatment goals: improvement and setting up of a maintenance program. The sequence of short-term goals outlined above measures improvement. During the process of developing the Part B guidelines, another form of treatment began to emerge. In Medicare terms, the federal government will pay for setting up a maintenance program, but not for carrying out a maintenance program. Setting up a home program is a good example. Treatment goals that ensure safety in a long-term care situation are covered by Medicare.

Maintenance programs, custodial care, and long-term care are health care needs that are excluded from Medicare coverage and most private insurance policies. The governmental provision of extended care has been the traditional responsibility of the states. The deinstitutionalization of state hospital patients took away the provision of most extended care. Therapists can identify a need for extended care, but very few therapists are employed by institutions that are mandated to provide it.

Step 5   The timing of long-term and short-term treatment goals is addressed in step 5. The clinical judgment of the therapist is tested by the need to prioritize and sequence treatment methods. A synthesis of the first 5 steps is required. As treatment progresses, there is a high probability that new information will require a different synthesis with different goals. At this point therapists should note that treatment begins with a mere sketch of a lot of information. Revisions are to be expected. If you seldom revise your treatment goals, you may be missing the implications of new information you discover during treatment. Changes in the frequency and duration of treatment, as well as in the treatment goals themselves, should be fairly common.

The first 5 steps of the documentation process may be summarized in the initial note. A tremendous amount of thought, clinical experience, and knowledge is required to set good treatment goals. The part of practice that needs to be strengthened is negotiating treatment goals with patients and caregivers. The activities are selected by the patients and caregivers. The quality of functional outcome is predicted by the therapist.

Step 6   Getting into the daily notations and weekly progress notes is a relief after the complex thought required to establish goals. The relief often expresses itself through a natural tendency to avoid changing goals. The easiest goal change occurs when a patient has a period of illness and needs to be placed on hold until he or she is well enough to participate in treatment again. Administrative pressures help us remember to avoid duplicating services and make sure that services are covered. The most difficult error to correct is an inaccurate prediction of what the patient will be able to achieve as a result of our services. An error suggests that the therapist must go back to the treatment planning process and think the whole thing over again. Go back to the initial note and try to find the source of the error. Consult another therapist. When you come up with a new goal to try, be candid in your documentation.

Reassessments and changes in goals are expected. You only look foolish when you adhere rigidly to a goal that is obviously not working, and reimbursement for useless services should be denied. Experience in working with a population is a great help in the early detection of a need to adjust treatment goals.

The design of a maintenance program is also recommended at step 6. Therapists often let this go until the day of discharge. More time is required to instruct the patient and caregiver and to iron out difficulties encountered after a period of use. A home program should be checked for safety and effectiveness, which is a reimbursable part of the stabilization process. An inability to generalize from the treatment setting to the discharge setting should also be addressed (Allen & Earhart, 1992).

Step 7   The monthly summary is a formal reexamination of the treatment goals (step 7). The long-term goals may need to be renegotiated with the patient and the caregiver, and a treatment session that is devoted to conducting another interview is a good idea that is seldom seen in current practice. The relationship between long-term goals and short-term goals should also be reexamined at this time. Medical reviewers expect to see necessary adjustments in the monthly summaries. Practicing therapists tend to see monthly summaries as a boring rehash of what they have already done, which is incorrect. Flexibility in adjusting services to the unique needs of the patient and the person's place in life is what is required. By requiring a monthly summary, the insurance industry is recognizing the time that a therapist needs to sit down and think. Use this time to organize your thoughts about this patient and improve your predictions of functional outcomes.

Step 8   The discharge summary helps you to benefit from your experience in working with this patient (step 8). The patient's record should identify the factors that contributed to or acted as barriers to treatment effectiveness. Barriers may include medical complications, lack of social or economic support, lack of commitment to change in a requested activity, or an inability to accept a disability. The reverse may also be true in that the factors contribute to effectiveness. Therapists should make a note of these impacts on treatment for future referral criteria and changes in treatment methods.

Documentation explains the importance of occupational therapy services. Steps 2 and 3 of this clinical reasoning process outline a way to think aboutmeaningful functional outcomes that help people adjust to the realities of living with a disability. Therapists will probably have to repeat these steps several times during the treatment process. The point is that steps 2 and 3 are frequently skipped in current practice. Therapists often jump in at step 4, with lengthy evaluations of measurable problems. The relationships between these problems, remaining abilities, and activity performance require more thought.

What a problem means to the individual and his or her social support system takes on a sense of significance during activity performance. Occupational therapy documentation should tell individual stories about changes in activity performance. I have yet to see a form or checklist that can capture the essence of what we do. A simple, short narrative note that tells a story about activities can let our readers understand what we do.

Do not be fooled by the words *simple* and *short*. To write simply and concisely is not easy or quick; it is the most difficult form of writing. Try writing a monthly summary that is one paragraph long that any high school graduate could understand. Several drafts will probably be required to eliminate information that may be valuable to you, but that your readers do not need or understand. This clinical reasoning process is designed to help you find and keep track of your major points.

The challenge of explaining the value of occupational therapy services is addressed in this chapter. These explanations may be improved by a clinical reasoning process that keeps the therapist's attention focused on making meaningful improvements in activity performance.

Reference   Allen, C.K., & Earhart, C.A. (1992). *Occupational therapy treatment goals for cognitive and physical disabilities.* Rockville, MD: American Occupational Therapy Association.

Figure 5.1 Steps in clinical reasoning

Therapist's Long Term Goals

Where OT Documents	What the Therapist Thinks!	What the Therapist Does!	What the Therapist Documents!
Step 1	**Step 1**	**Step 1**	**Step 1**
Initial note	Rely on previous knowledge and experience regarding diagnosis and problems Make judgments in response to observations	Literature review as needed Review MD orders and medical record and/or speak with referral service Observes patient	Primary diagnosis Treatment diagnosis Date of onset Written physician order Record prior functional level/history Record whether patient has been treated by OT previously <u>Outcome</u> Predict Natural Course of Disease
Step 2	**Step 2**	**Step 2**	**Step 2**
Initial note	Determine interview/evaluation format	Interview: Patient Patient & Caregiver or Caregiver only Obtain patient/caregiver goals	Record patient/caregiver goals and available social, economic, and physical supports <u>Outcome</u> Request for activities—along with available social-economic support

ΛΟΤΛ

The American Occupational Therapy Association, Inc.

1383 Piccard Drive P.O. Box 1725
Rockville, MD 20850-4375

Figure 5.1 (continued)

Therapist's Long-Term Goals and Changes in Goals

Where OT Documents	What the Therapist Thinks!	What the Therapist Does!	What the Therapist Documents!
Step 3	Step 3	Step 3	Step 3
A. Initial note	A. Analyze physical and cognitive abilities required to do requested activities	A. Do quick assessment of physical and cognitive activities Screen physical and cognitive	A. Record quick assessment
	B. Make initial hypothesis about underlying factors affecting function Begin to formulate problem list	B. Observe performance of requested activity	B. Record patient's baseline dysfunctional performance in requested activities
	C. Decide whether further evaluation is indicated Yes ____ No ____ If yes, which evaluation tools will be used	C. Evaluate patient using selected instruments	C. Record underlying evaluation results: physical, cognitive, environmental
	D. Estimate Long-Term Goals (LTGs) • Cognitive Abilities • Physical Abilities • Social & Physical Supports • Natural Course of the Disease	D. Verify goals with patient/caregiver	D. Record rehabilitation potential in requested activities, which is the long-term goal

**The American
Occupational Therapy
Association, Inc.**

1383 Piccard Drive P.O. Box 1725
Rockville, MD 20850-4375

Figure 5.1 (continued)

Therapist's Short-Term Goals and Changes in Goals

Where OT Documents	What the Therapist Thinks!	What the Therapist Does!	What the Therapist Documents!
Step 4	Step 4	Step 4	Step 4
2nd part of initial note	A. Sequence short-term goals (STGs) to: • meet needs and wants of patient • according to the progression of recovery B. Select treatment plans to: • reduce pain • prevent accidents/injuries • make neuromuscular changes • compensate for physical or cognitive disabilities • teach substitutions • monitor sparing • monitor recovery	Establish baseline measures for STGs	Record STGs and expected sequence Record baseline measures
Step 5	Step 5	Step 5	Step 5
	Estimate frequency and duration of treatment Consider family and other caregivers who provide assistance	Explain the relationship between LTGs and STGs and treatment planning to patient caregivers Teach assistive techniques to family and caregivers Check estimates of frequency, duration and degree with other members of the treatment plan	Record expected relationship between short-term and long-term goals and the therapist's treatment plan Record assistive techniques to family & caregivers Record expected frequency, duration and degree for obtainment of STGs and LTGs

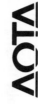

The American Occupational Therapy Association, Inc.

1383 Piccard Drive P.O. Box 1725
Rockville, MD 20850-4375

Figure 5.1 (continued)

Therapist's Short-Term Goals and Changes in Goals

Where OT Documents	What the Therapist Thinks!	What the Therapist Does!	What the Therapist Documents!
Step 6	**Step 6**	**Step 6**	**Step 6**

• Daily notations on chart
• Weekly progress note
• Monthly summary notes
	Constantly re-assessing goals:
	  • Are treatment services covered?
	  • Are you duplicating services and
	
	  and
	
	Are you providing maintenance care?
	
	  and
	
	Are you changing plans as necessary?
	and also consider:
	  • Should patient be put on hold for a period of time due to illness?
	  • Do you need to design a maintenance program for residual deficits?
		• Chart review
		• Provide treatment
		• Observe performance in requested activities
		• Modify treatment according to patient's response to STG & LTG
		
		As patient goals change you modify treatment
		  • Verify new short-term and long-term goals with patient/caregivers
		  • Discontinue patient temporarily
		  • Instruct in-home program
			• Record briefly:
			  Date, type, length of treatment
			• State change in meeting short-term goals and the effect on long-term goals
			• Record changes in goals in weekly or monthly notes
			• Every 30 days summarize changes in patient's ability to perform functional activities and changes in underlying factors
			• State when patient reaches goals. Explanation if patient does not reach goals and and how that affects treatment plan
			• Recertification of Medicare
			• Record temporary discontinuation of treatment and reason
			• Record home program and any follow-up recommendations made

ΛΟΤΛ

The American
Occupational Therapy
Association, Inc.

1383 Piccard Drive P.O. Box 1725
Rockville, MD 20850-4375

Figure 5.1 (continued)

Therapist's Evaluation of Treatment Effectiveness

Where OT Documents	What the Therapist Thinks!	What the Therapist Does!	What the Therapist Documents!
Step 7	**Step 7**	**Step 7**	**Step 7**
Monthly summary	Re-examine estimated LTGs for requested activities Re-examine relationship between LTGs and STGs	Make note for future LTGs Make note for future LTGs & STGs and treatment plans	Record degree of attainment of LTGs Record strength of association in meeting LTGs and STGs and treatment plans
Step 8	**Step 8**	**Step 8**	**Step 8**
Discharge Summary	Consider other factors that are barriers to treatment: • medical complications • lack of social or economic supports • lack of commitment to change in requested activities • unable to accept disability Consider other factors that contributed to treatment effectiveness. • social & economic support • commitment to change • functional history	Make note for future referral criteria	Record other factors that contributed to or acted as barriers to treatment effectiveness

ΛΟΤΛ

The American Occupational Therapy Association, Inc.

1383 Piccard Drive P.O. Box 1725
Rockville, MD 20850-4375

6. Reports That Work

Mary Foto, OTR, FAOTA
Claudia Allen, MA, OTR, FAOTA
Caroline Bass, OTR
Terry Moon-Sperling, OTR
Dorothy Wilson, OTR, FAOTA
in consultation with
Suzanne Robben Brown, MPH, PT

This chapter originally appeared as Issue 9 of the AOTA Self-Study Series: Assessing Function. *The authors have a unique perspective since they have worked with third party payers on reimbursement for occupational therapy services. They have important information to share regarding the best way to document services.*

Mary Foto is a senior allied health consultant, Blue Cross of California, Van Nuys, CA.

Claudia Allen is an occupational therapy consultant, Blue Cross of California, Van Nuys, CA.

Caroline Bass is an occupational therapy consultant, Blue Cross of California, Van Nuys, CA.

Terry Moon-Sperling is an occupational therapy consultant, Blue Cross of California, Van Nuys, CA.

Dorothy Wilson is an occupational therapy consultant, Blue Cross of California, Van Nuys, CA.

Suzanne Robben Brown is director and assistant professor, physical therapy department, Langston University, OK. She is also president of Health*Wise, Inc., a rehabilitation consulting firm.

$\mathbf{D}$ocumentation of occupational therapy services provides a legal and clinical record for reimbursement. The occupational therapy assessment report is written for those outside the occupational therapy profession. It is directed to physicians, health care administrators, attorneys, allied health professionals, insurance companies or payers, employers, and schools. One cannot assume, therefore, that those reading the occupational therapy reports are familiar with the theoretical base or subsequent use of *Occupational Therapy Uniform Terminology—2nd Edition* (AOTA, 1989). Yet each report must communicate the unique ability of occupational therapists to assess impairment, disability, and handicap.

A primary reason for developing report writing skills in today's health care system is to secure payment for services rendered. Unless health care delivery institutions are adequately reimbursed for occupational therapy services, these institutions will not be able to justify continuing providing occupational therapy services on a timely basis or sufficient scale to affect a patient's outcome. The basis for payment decisions by third party payers is your occupational therapy report in the patient's clinical record.

Occupational therapy reports also offer legal evidence of reasonable action and intervention. Many therapists respond by offering copious records of routine actions, yet often do not document the clinical reasoning behind the actions and the subsequent response. Complete records written in a clear, concise, and direct style convey valued professional judgment and are the best legal defense against the threat of lawsuit.

A patient's clinical record of occupational therapy services is the document from which conclusions are drawn about the patient's impairment, disability, or handicap. It documents the relationship between assessment and intervention and establishes the relevance and justification for referral and subsequent treatment. Information presented in each occupational therapy report should be selected and synthesized carefully. It is not necessary to include all clinical information gathered in a patient's permanent written record.

Although each practice setting dictates specific requirements for documentation and report writing, several general principles of data collection and presentation apply to all settings. Medical payment standards have evolved from legal and government requirements and are reflected in standards for medical documentation. For example, it is a legal requirement to sign and date any therapy report. Because of this requirement, most government agencies and medical facilities also require each therapist to sign and date *all* documentation.

The medical payment standards identified here reflect requirements applicable throughout the United States. Medicare documentation and report requirements are cited most often owing to their impact on the entire health care services industry. However, local custom, requirements, and policies may take precedence over these guidelines in certain instances. For example, the Joint Commission on the Accreditation of Healthcare Organizations (JCAHO) requires biweekly progress notes for patients in a rehabilitation setting, while the facility may require weekly progress notes.

Occupational therapy records must meet the requirements of more than one industry—for example, private insurance, worker's compensation, state or government regulatory agencies, and the personal injury legal system. All request or require occupational therapy records.

In this chapter, we address three specific types of occupational therapy reports: (1) occupational therapy assessment reports, (2) treatment plans, and (3) progress reports. The assessment report is the report specifically written for those outside the occupational therapy profession. The treatment plan and progress report formats are used as supportive documents to the assessment report and within one's facility to report treatment activity and patient status. These three report formats compose a comprehensive record of occupational therapy services, and the guidelines suggested reflect the current industry standards.

Principles of Documentation

Before discussing each type of occupational therapy report, we present four principles of documentation. These principles are the foundation for all successful occupational therapy reports because they enable you to communicate both the patient's status as well as your professional expertise.

Principle #1

Terms used in occupational therapy reports must be accepted by the target audience.

The occupational therapy assessment report interprets the occupational therapy evaluation for outside agencies. In assessment reports, and the supplemental treatment plans and progress reports, use language that is readily understood by your target audience.

Avoid occupational therapy jargon; use it only in your treatment or daily notes. When you use occupational therapy terminology (i.e., from the *Uniform Terminology for Occupational Therapy— 2nd Edition*) to convey patient status, you need to explain these terms to your audience or you open the possibility for misinterpretation and an incorrect or negative review (AOTA, 1989).

Identify the terms accepted by the industry to which you are directing your reports. Two examples follow.

Example 1
- "The patient is unable to don shoes secondary to deficit in sensory motor performance components." (Occupational therapy terminology.)
- "The patient is unable to put on shoes due to lack of sitting balance." (Industry-accepted terminology.)

Example 2
- "The patient has moderate-to-severe perceptual deficits." (Occupational therapy terminology.)

- "The patient is unable to locate the right sleeve hole when putting on his shirt." (Industry-accepted terminology.)

Medical terms and ratings that have been accepted by both the casualty insurance and legal industries are found in the American Medical Association's *Guides for the Evaluation of Permanent Impairment* for worker's compensation and personal injury cases (AMA, 1984). The *Guide* uses range of motion and disability ratings pertinent to occupational therapy. It has been accepted by several states, which have used it when writing their state legal codes.

Accepted terms for functional assistance levels are published in the *Medicare Hospital Manual* Outpatient Occupational Therapy Medicare Part B Guidelines (DHHS Transmittal No. 565) for medical review of Medicare providers.

Specialized practice settings may have their own accepted terms and definitions, but these should only be used in a therapist's treatment notes for that setting.

Principle #2   *Concepts* used in occupational therapy reports must be translated to a wide audience.

The use of concepts and selection of words in written reports frequently reflects a school of thought or a theoretical model. For example, "The child's vestibular activity is severely depressed, causing problems in his/her visual comprehension," reflects the theoretical sensory integration model. Be careful. Although it is important for you to base your clinical case on comprehensive theoretical constructs, these concepts may not be adequately understood beyond the world of specialized practitioners. In developing an assessment report, use easily understood terms that highlight the appropriateness of both your professional assessment and treatment plan.

Principle #3   Occupational therapy reports must be appropriate both in terms of writing style and *editorial intent*.

The manner by which thoughts are conveyed in writing is called *style*. This includes grammar and composition, word usage, and format. The writing of all occupational therapists should reflect professional standards: correct English grammar, logic, and syntax; complete and well-composed sentences; and composition in a form that is logical, coherent, and concise. Style that reflects professional standards helps the reader understand your evaluation.

Industries to which occupational therapy reports are directed expect that the patients will be evaluated in one of two ways: in terms of *abilities* (positive attributes) or in terms of *deficits* (negative attributes). These attributes are documented through editorial intent. Some examples are:

- "Patient is *able* to dress upper body independently, requires assistance for lower extremities." (Positive)
- "Patient is *unable* to dress self independently." (Negative)

- "Patient is able to prepare a light snack with sequencing and following safety precautions." (Positive)
- "Patient is unable to cut meat." (Negative)
- "Patient is able to feed self after full set up." (Positive)
- "Patient requires minimal assistance to feed self." (Negative)

Your presentation of the editorial intent should be determined by the industry requesting documentation of occupational therapy services. For example, an employer requesting an occupational therapy evaluation of an employee will expect an abilities assessment—that is, what can this employee do. A request from an employee's lawyer may be for a "deficits assessment"—that is, what can't this employee do. The problems identified in the treatment plan are always listed as deficits.

Also, Medicare requires that editorial intent convey functional deficits. Knowing what your reader expects to receive and how it will be used helps you write effective occupational therapy reports.

Principle #4   Occupational therapy reports must use a standardized reporting format.

The format most commonly seen in medical documentation is a *structured narrative* report. How the narrative is structured is dependent upon local custom, facility policy, and/or purpose of the report.

An assessment report is one example of a structured narrative. It is structured to include the following sections in order: introduction, physical findings, and interpretation of findings, followed by the treatment plan. This format is appropriate for a wide audience and should be used when reports are to be distributed outside your facility, to physicians, or to legal entities (i.e., courts or employers). All reports should be typewritten, single spaced with double space between paragraphs. A sample narrative report is given in Figure 6.1.

Note how this sample assessment report and treatment plan follow the three documentation principles. This well-written occupational therapy report highlights both the patient's status and the occupational therapist's clinical reasoning. It is clear, uses simple language, and is presented in a logical and easy-to-follow format.

Another reporting format used in occupational therapy is the *SOAP format.* The structure is: subjective, objective, assessment findings and treatment plan. This format is a modification of the Problem-Oriented Medical Record (POMR) as developed by Weed (1971), which has four sections: a database, problem list, treatment plan, and SOAP or progress notes.

The SOAP format is best used for communicating treatment notes or daily documentation within and between facilities. It is not appropriate for professional correspondence that is intended to convey your clinical reasoning and justify occupational therapy intervention.

Figure 6.1 Sample assessment report and treatment plan

Introduction

J. is a 53-year-old male who suffered a right CVA 5 weeks prior to referral. He is being referred to OT to maximize his independence in activities of daily living. J. lives with his wife and his preschool-age grand-daughter in a single-story home. Prior to the stroke, he was in good health and was recently retired from his job as a retail store operator. J. was treated in an acute facility for 6 days and then transferred to a rehabilita-tion unit where he received daily occupational and physical therapy and was discharged in a wheelchair, requiring minimum assistance for basic self-care activities.

Physical Findings

J.'s wife is in good health and, since J.'s retirement, shares responsibility for watching their grandchild during the day with J. She volunteers one day a week at their church luncheon and has expressed concern about J.'s ability to safely prepare a hot lunch for himself and his granddaughter. She states that J. some-times forgets to turn off the stove and cannot safely regulate the flames of their gas range. A cold lunch would be acceptable to J.'s wife, J., and his grandchild if he could manage independently or with the wife's minimum assistance before she leaves or with help by the grandchild. J. is unable to prepare a cold meal without moderate assistance at this time. He is unable to stand to retrieve dishes from the cabinet without falling to his right side. His dominant left upper extremity becomes a tightly held fist and bent at the elbow when he attempts to reach for objects. J. ignores obstacles in the path of his wheelchair that are located on his left side and frequently has to be reminded of the next step in an activity before he can proceed.

Interpretation of Findings

In my professional opinion, J. requires skilled OT to alleviate the problems that make him unable to pre-pare a meal without assistance. Occupational therapy intervention is needed to increase J.'s standing balance to prevent falling and injury. Skilled therapy is also required to control the increased flexor tone that interferes with J.'s use of his left upper extremity for reaching and carrying objects. J. and J.'s wife need to be instructed in techniques to control the flexor tone and compensate for the left-side neglect and apraxia demonstrated during attempts to prepare a meal. The goal agreed to by J. and J.'s wife is minimum assistance for cold meal preparation in 3 weeks. J. has good rehabilitation potential to achieve each of these goals.

Treatment Plan

Problem: Unsafe meal preparation.

Goals: Occupational therapy will: increase standing balance 50%, control left upper extremity flexor tone for effective grasp and release during forward reach, and increase J.'s ability to remember all steps required to prepare a meal so that J. will be able to prepare a cold lunch after set-up of items by his wife.

Intervention:

    1. Meal preparation activities.
    2. Activities to improve tone in the left upper extremity.
    3. Dynamic standing activities.
    4. Instruct wife regarding safety hazards and compensation techniques.

Frequency: 3 times per week.

Duration: 3 weeks.

_____ Signature

Within a facility, occupational therapists can use the SOAP format to structure the collection of clinical data to be used later in more formal reports.

This format is used to record initial evaluation data as well as subsequent progress. It is appropriate for facilities in which a common clinical record is maintained or where frequent short notations are required or communication occurs across disciplines. SOAP format entries are frequently made in outline form, using abbreviations and professional jargon to record information. Effective communication in this format requires that both the writer and the reader be familiar with the format. A sample SOAP note is given in Figure 6.2.

Figure 6.2 Sample SOAP note

Subjective—Automatic speech echolalia.

Objective—Seen to increase self-feeding and swallowing independence. Continues with restorative feeding program and ate 20% of meal. May try bolus feedings to facilitate return of appetite.

Assessment—Moderate assist for feeding is due to distractibility/fatigue and initiation apraxis. Moderate dysphagia with delayed swallow, manipulation of bolus posteriorly. Moderate increased tone in R elbow interferes with ability to bring food to mouth using dominate RUE. Improvement continues with right labial closure (minimal spillage).

Plan—Continue self-feeding/swallow retraining. Consider orthosis to inhibit tone of Right elbow.

Notice how the SOAP report format makes use of jargon and a shorthand of medical, technical terms, and observations that may be unfamiliar to a reader outside the facility or profession.

Occupational Therapy Reports

The occupational therapy patient record is made up of a series of occupational therapy documents. Three reports included in this patient record are written for those outside your facility: assessment report, treatment plans, and progress reports. Each of these reports is discussed separately below. The accepted formats of medical report writing that are presented will allow you to demonstrate the clinical reasoning that underpins your occupational therapy practice.

Occupational Therapy Assessment Report

The patient information collected in an occupational therapy assessment serves many purposes. The database of information is used for planning treatment, setting goals, predicting recovery and outcome, and measuring progress. The occupational therapy assessment report is the interpretation of this database.

A well-structured assessment report is divided into three major sections: the introduction, physical findings, and the interpretation of findings. Although some sections may appear more important to you, as the clinician, than others, it is important to your audience to follow the structured narrative format, with findings noted in the appropriate sections. If there are no findings or the information cannot be obtained, be sure to indicate this.

Introduction

A patient's current medical and functional condition is summarized in the introduction. This information is obtained from an interview with the patient and his or her family and from a review of pertinent medical charts. The summary should include the evaluation date, patient identifying information, referral information, and a review of the patient's history.

Evaluation date. This evaluation date may presented as on the written record or stated in the opening sentence of the report (e.g., "Thelma Jones was seen on November 29, 1988 for . . .").

Patient identifying information. The name, age, and sex of the patient should be written out fully. To facilitate reimbursement and medical review, use the name as it appears on the financial record or insurance card.

Referral information. The source and purpose of the referral and the medical diagnosis should be stated. Include in this statement the primary functional area requiring occupational therapy intervention (e.g., ". . . is referred by Dr. Fixit for assessment of activities of daily living" or "The family requests occupational therapy assessment.").

Most third party payers—and Medicare, in particular—require a medical diagnosis. Uniform codes for medical diagnoses are given in the *International Classification of Diseases, 9th Ed.*, (ICD-9) Manual. Use these codes when citing diagnoses.

The presentation of your information will vary depending on the relationship between the medical diagnosis and your occupational therapy diagnosis. If the medical diagnosis and relevant diagnosis for occupational therapy are the same, state this after the reason for referral. Relevant diagnoses indicate a recognized pathology or impairment that requires occupational therapy intervention (e.g., hemiplegia, cerebral palsy, schizophrenia, or closed head injury.)

If the medical diagnosis *contributes* to the impairment but does not describe the impairment, present the information as medical history (e.g., "Thelma Jones, 45-year-old female, is referred for assessment of home management activities. The patient has a history of diabetes mellitus with neuropathies.").

History. Medical, functional, vocational, and family history and previous rehabilitation care should be noted if they are relevant to the patient's current functional status. Medical history should include references to previous illnesses, surgery, or injury involving the same body system(s) for the same condition within the previous 5 years.

Functional history should include previous functional level, and socioeconomic, educational, and residential status. Highest functional level ever achieved and most recent functional status should be included in all assessment reports. This information may be helpful in predicting the patient's potential for rehabilitation or explaining his or her response to treatment. Socioeconomic information, including information about family or other caregivers that suggests resource constraints or exceptional resource availability, should be included.

Vocational and recreational histories are helpful in corroborating the highest and most recent levels of function. Family history should be noted when there is evidence of related genetic or hereditary disease in order to anticipate the course of the disease and its potential effect on the intervention you propose.

Your presentation of the patient's history should be direct and concise. All information should be selected carefully in terms of its relevance to setting treatment goals, selecting the treatment plan, and predicting the potential for rehabilitation. If there is no relevant history, state this in the introduction (e.g., "History relevant to the patient's problem is not significant").

Note any previous occupational therapy received for the current condition or related conditions. Also include concurrent rehabilitation therapies, such as physical or speech therapy, psychological support or counseling, or vocational retraining. Indicate if the patient has not received any previous occupational therapy for the present condition.

Physical Findings
The aim of occupational therapy is to make improvements in functional activities that are meaningful to the patients and their caregivers.

The physical findings section of the assessment report should begin with a statement of the activities that the patient and caregiver identify as problematic and needing improvement. These functional disabilities are then used to establish a request for services that can be targeted to construct a meaningful examination. Your documentation will serve to establish baseline functional disability and provide the objective measurements for charting.

The classic definition of *physical findings* derives from the field of medicine in which physical findings are the results of tests and measurements (AMA, 1984). In occupational therapy, functional activity is the measure for physical findings. The activity to be measured must, therefore, be selected carefully because these activities are used to justify the value of occupational therapy services.

A selected activity must:

- be meaningful to the patient and caregiver.
- be recognized as medically necessary.
- have potential for improvement.

Regarding third party payers, Medicare, for example, recognizes the importance of self-care tasks in the activities of daily living, but work and play/leisure activities are not covered. However, *safety* in play/leisure activities can be covered due to medical necessity. The best justification for occupational therapy services is a recommended activity with descriptions of safety precautions that require specialized assistance to prevent further injury.

The description of your findings should follow each selected activity. The physical findings should include the level of assistance required to complete the activity safely. Brief statements describing amount of physical or cognitive assistance, task sequence, and structure requirements are useful.

Performance component data (for example, underlying physical and cognitive factors) in the assessment report minimize the value of occupational therapy services. It is recommended that you do not continue this practice. Instead, adopt the format and content suggested above and present the information in a style that makes the value of occupational therapy readily apparent. Record performance components in your treatment or daily notes.

Interpretation of Findings
Clinical reasoning is conveyed through the synthesis of data on a patient's medical condition and functional deficits and is reflected in the therapist's request for services, physical findings, and expected rate of improvement.

It is the interpretation section of the assessment report that is used most often by medical reviewers and payers to establish the need for occupational therapy services. Your presentation and choice of words is therefore critical in ensuring proper medical review and reimbursement.

Medical reviewers determine the medical necessity for care and the need for skilled (professional) care. When documenting the need for service, do not assume that a reviewer will understand the medical necessity for care or your professional judgment as an occupational therapist. Both must be stated clearly at the beginning of the interpretation of findings section. Two standard statements are:

1. "In my professional opinion, this patient requires skilled occupational therapy because . . ." and

2. "In my professional opinion, this patient's condition requires occupational therapy care due to . . ."

    Follow this statement with:

    - a summary of abnormal findings presented in the history and physical findings sections.
    - a concise statement of the patient's functional deficits (impairments, disabilities, or handicaps).
    - the expected improvement or compensation to result from occupational therapy (e.g., therapy goals).
    - any unusual precautions or contradictions arising from the patient's medical status (routine precautions covered by normal policies and procedures do not need to be stated).

In occupational therapy reports for Medicare, conclude your interpretation section with a statement regarding "rehabilitation potential." We have found therapists at times have difficulty with the concept of rehabilitation potential. Rehabilitation potential is defined as the therapist's and/or physician's expectation concerning the patient's ability to meet the goals at the initiation of treatment. You must therefore state therapy goals that the patient will achieve and not reference your patient's goals to "normal" function. Your determination of a patient's rehabilitation potential has important consequences for reimbursement. If you complete the interpretation section as suggested—that is, reporting functional deficits that are expected to improve as a result of occupational therapy services—your Medicare patient will have "good" rehabilitation potential for the expected outcome or therapy goals stated.

Your presentation of clear, complete, and concise interpretation statements is very important in demonstrating your clinical reasoning as a professional occupational therapist, the rationale for treatment, and the basis for reimbursement. Practice writing such statements.

Treatment Plan

A treatment plan documents what you will do (your intervention) to improve the functional activity level of your patient. Having well-formed goals is critical to a successful treatment plan.

A treatment plan should report the following:

- problems
- goals
- specific intervention (methods)
- frequency/duration of treatment

This list includes the minimum requirements by Medicare. Your plan should reflect the clinical data documented in the assessment report.

Depending on the policy of your facility, your treatment plan may be a separate document from your assessment report. Having a separate report allows a reviewer or payer to scan the proposed treatment for a patient quickly, review the treatment to date, and monitor progress without having to read a patient's entire clinical record.

The treatment plan should be updated continuously as patients progress through their course of treatment. Goals should be revised as in the following example:

> The initial goal is to improve upper body dressing by increasing shoulder flexion range of motion to 90 degrees. The revised goal now includes increasing flexor strength to a grade of 4 minus to achieve the desired functional outcome.

By updating your treatment plan regularly, you will demonstrate continuity of care, patient's progress, and reflect your decision-making skill in response to your patient's needs.

Problems

The problems to be addressed through intervention should be stated precisely, as few people read the treatment notes and more read the treatment plan. Remember that problems are stated in negative terms and referred to as functional performance deficits.

Goals

Treatment goals are what the patient and/or caregiver will do—that is, *their* expected accomplishments. Occupational therapy enables the patient or caregiver to achieve each of these goals. The resolution of a patient problem should be identified in the goals (e.g., "Patient achieved goal of independent lower body dressing").

Goal statements have two parts: the functional outcome statement and the enabling intent. A functional outcome statement identifies the desired patient performance resulting from therapy. Activities selected in the physical findings section of the assessment report should be referenced with the desired level of assistance.

Enabling intent clarifies or identifies the method by which a therapist enables a patient to accomplish the stated goal (e.g., improvement in specific activity or in performance components; sensory motor integration, neuromuscular or motor performance, cognitive level, or psychological skills). Examples of functional outcome/ enabling goal statements are:

- "Occupational therapy will increase upper extremity strength (strength grade—good) [enabling intent] sufficient to allow the patient to be independent in dressing activities [functional outcome]."
- "Occupational therapy will increase range of motion of right shoulder (30%) [enabling intent] sufficient to allow patient to reach kitchen cupboards at shoulder level [functional outcome]."
- "Occupational therapy will attain adequate sequencing ability [enabling intent] to allow meal preparation by the patient with minimal verbal assistance of the caregiver [functional outcome]."

Goals should be specific to the time a patient is within a particular setting (e.g., during a patient's stay in an acute rehabilitation setting, during a specified period of home health care). Goals should not overlap practice settings.

Specific Interventions (Methods)

The interventions and methods proposed and used must be specified for each goal and stated clearly in the treatment plan.

Frequency/Duration of Treatment

Statements on the frequency and duration of treatment should include the number of visits per defined time period (usually stated in weeks or months). Base your estimate of the frequency and duration of treatment on recognized norms or recovery curves for the patient's impairment, disability, or handicap. Any conditions or environmental factors expected to increase the normally expected frequency or duration must be stated clearly.

Progress Reports

Documentation of patient progress serves as evidence to substantiate payment or appropriateness of the care (quality assurance).

After you have completed your initial assessment report and treatment plan, you are ready to begin the intervention and monitor your patient's progress. Several types of documents are used by occupational therapists to compile or record subsequent progress:

- treatment notes
- progress notes
- progress summary report
- discharge summary report

Each type of document has a specific purpose and identified content. The link between the treatment plan and the progress summary report are a series of treatment and progress notes. These notes comprise documentation that may be required for reimbursement but only as a supplement to the formal written assessment report, treatment plan, and progress summary report. When used together, these documents provide content to substantiate both the progress achieved through the occupational therapy intervention and the need for continued skilled care.

Treatment Notes

Treatment notes are also called "daily notes." These are brief written entries to document services provided to a patient according to your treatment plan. They should be written each time a patient is seen or scheduled for treatment. In fact, some type of notation for each treatment is required by payers to verify that care was provided. Treatment notes also serve as a record of change in patient's status, leading to a modified treatment plan. They are not, however, a comprehensive assessment of patient's progress and therefore do not constitute an occupational therapy report.

When writing treatment notes, include at a minimum:

- date of service
- type of service
- specific problem(s) treated
- patient response
- therapist signature

You may also wish to include other appropriate information, such as:

- educational information given to the patient
- changes in physical, mental, socioeconomic, or caregiver status
- physician visits or other medical treatment
- receipt of special equipment or adaptive aids
- critical incidents (falls, burns, unusual pains)
- precautions taken during treatment specific to the patient's individual needs

Flow charts are useful to document treatment notes rather than separate entries in a narrative or SOAP note format. The flow chart should provide space for listing of the separate components of the treatment plan, daily listings for treatments performed (checkmark areas), provider's initials daily, and a full signature area to identify initials. Additional space on the bottom of the form or the reverse side for written comments should be provided and used.

Progress Notes

Progress notes are required by many outside agencies and are reviewed as essential building blocks to the formal progress summary report. They summarize a series of treatment notes and reflect clinical reasoning by modification of the treatment plan. Because they are a record of your clinical reasoning, they should only be written by you, the occupational therapist, and not by other personnel.

How often you complete progress notes will depend on your practice setting. Acute care facilities may require progress notes to be written every other day, while inpatient rehabilitation facilities may produce weekly progress notes. Outpatient facilities may vary their requirements based on type of patient, while Medicare-approved outpatient facilities are required to complete progress notes weekly. Long-term facilities may only require monthly or even less frequent progress notes.

Regardless of the frequency, content of progress notes should include the patient's treatment, progress, and existing treatment plan. At a minimum, the progress note should contain:

- dates of treatments
- activities performed
- patient response
- goals achieved, problems remaining
- treatment plan modifications including discharge plans

Each progress note should start with the date and conclude with the therapist's signature.

To maintain continuity, the format for recording treatments performed and patient response should be the same as that used in your treatment notes, summarizing what has occurred during the time period involved. Avoid vague, noninformative statements, such as "Patient tolerated treatment well."

Goals should be stated the same way as in your treatment plan. As the patient progresses, you will develop and report new goals and modify your treatment plan as appropriate. Progress achieved during the time period involved often appears more significant when stated in a weekly progress note than in daily treatment notes. If reimbursement for care depends on regular progress, then you will want to state clearly the cumulative progress achieved over time in your progress notes, emphasizing the deficits remaining.

Progress Summary Reports

Progress summary reports are reevaluations of your treatment plan and progress notes. A progress summary report documents a therapist's evaluation and interpretation, as well as the patient's achievement.

Progress summaries are commonly used to determine the need for continued care and payment for care. Because of their nature, these progress summaries should always be written by a licensed therapist.

How often progress summaries are written depends on their use. Progress summaries written for physicians, for example, are prepared in advance of a patient's return appointment, while progress summaries written for third party payers are submitted with each billing statement. Progress summary reports prepared by therapists working in acute or ambulatory care settings are usually written every 30 days, while those for long-term settings are usually written every 3 months.

Regardless of their frequency, all progress summaries should be written clearly and in a format similar to the initial assessment report. Each progress summary should include at a minimum:

- length of time patient has been treated
- treatments received, amount, and types
- current physical findings and functional performance levels
- patient response to treatments
- progress since last summary or evaluation
- changes in treatment plan
- discharge planning activities
- prognosis for the next treatment period
- need for continued skilled care

By including the length of time a patient has been treated and the amount and types of treatments, a reviewer can establish the severity of the patient's condition and the effectiveness of the treatment plan. If the treatment plan has been modified, an explanation should be offered relating to the expected outcome or goals. If a separate treatment plan is used, attach the updated plan to the progress summary. Reporting discharge planning activities, such as presentation of a home program, obtaining adaptive equipment, referral to medical or community resources, and patient/family education activities, demonstrates your encouragement of a patient's independence from continuing care. Discharge planning activities should be evident from the start of occupational therapy services. As in your initial assessment reports for Medicare patients, include a statement of rehabilitation potential, expected frequency of treatment, and duration of the total care. Figures 6.3, 6.4, and 6.5 present samples of three different types of progress reporting documents: progress note, progress report, and discharge summary report.

Discharge Summary Reports

Discharge summary reports are a type of progress summary and should be written in the same style as that used for your initial assessment report and subsequent progress summaries. Include the following:

- introduction
- physical findings
- discharge plans
- activity assessment

Figure 6.3 Sample weekly progress note

3/24/89

The patient has attended 3 of 3 treatment sessions this past week with a total of 16 sessions since the initiation of occupational therapy. There has been an increased willingness to work with this therapist this past week, which may be attributed to the addition of a mild antidepressant 2 weeks ago. The focus this past week has been to increase independence with bathing and light meal preparation. The patient is now able to transfer into the tub using a transfer tub bench with standby assist of 1 person and bathe using a long-handled sponge, which has been issued to the patient. Sandwich preparation is done with verbal cuing to use the left upper extremity as a gross assist. Safety hazards are anticipated appropriately. Patient and husband continue to follow through with the home program of self range of motion and self-care activities. The patient's new goal is to be able to prepare a hot meal. Plan to decrease occupational therapy to 2 times per week to achieve this goal and anticipate discharge at the end of next week.

_____ OTR

Figure 6.4 Sample monthly progress report

6/30/89

The patient has been seen three times per week since 6/5/89 for the following program: seated and standing activities of daily living with appropriate equipment, functional upper extremity reeducation, home program and family instruction.

Progress includes decreased lability. The patient has been able to refrain from crying during therapy as she is now able to focus on her abilities rather than her deficits. The family also reports fewer crying sessions at home.

Previously, the patient was using a reacher to don pants over her feet but now uses the crossed leg technique without need for equipment. The patient was dependent for donning shoes but now dons the right shoe independently with velcro closures and the left shoe requires maximum assistance due to a tight fitting AFO. Upper extremity dressing is independent except for hooking her bra. Kitchen skills have improved from a dependent to independent cutting of food items with an adapted cutting board and rocker knife. Progress has been made from seated only activities to maintaining standing balance at the kitchen counter with minimal assistance while making a cake. The patient is now able to crack eggs and use an electric mixer with a one-handed technique. Patient has been issued a suction brush for washing dishes. The family has been observing good follow-through of these techniques at home.

Problems at this time include a nonfunctional left upper extremity due to flaccidity and pain with shoulder flexion and abduction beyond 70 degrees. Cues to position the flaccid left upper extremity prior to sitting are required due to the left side neglect.

PLAN: Continue occupational therapy treatment 3 times per week with the following goals:

1. Increase the use of the left upper extremity as a gross stabilizer through the facilitation of tone and techniques to incorporate the increased tone with functional activities.
2. Maintain safe balance independently while standing and performing activities of daily living, especially with meal preparation.
3. Patient will show improved left side awareness by positioning the left upper extremity prior to sitting.
4. The patient and the family will continue to follow through with the prescribed home program on a consistent basis.

The above plan has been discussed and agreed upon by the patient and family. Discharge from outpatient occupational therapy is anticipated to be on 8/11/89.

_____ OTR

Effective Documentation for Occupational Therapy

Figure 6.5   Sample discharge summary

9/29/89

Summary and Recommendations:

Mr. A. is a 78-year-old male, who on 6/4/89 suffered a CVA with left hemiparesis while on vacation in Florida. Past medical history includes adult onset diabetes mellitus and hypertension. A referral for occupational therapy was received on 8/7/89; however, it was not initiated until 8/25/89 due to the patient being hospitalized for a psychiatric illness. Mr. A. was seen 14 times from 8/25/89 to 10/30/89 at a frequency initially at 3 times per week, decreasing to once a week for the last week. Attendance was inconsistent due to problems with transportation that was provided by the family. There was poor family follow-through to utilize the available community resources for transportation.

Mr. A. initially presented with the following problems:

- Minimal to moderate assistance with activities of daily living skills (injecting insulin, bathing, dressing, feeding, cooking, performing housework) due to a moderate left side neglect, impulsive behavior, decreased safety awareness, and difficulty in sequencing the steps in the performance of a task.
- Decreased dynamic standing balance with the above activities.
- Nonfunctional left upper extremity (abnormal tone, decreased range of motion, painful shoulder, questionable voluntary movement).

Through adaptation and specialized instruction, the patient was able to independently use a one-handed lancing device for testing blood. The patient was referred to a diabetic education consultant, and it was found that monitoring of blood and insulin consumption was performed accurately and that further visits were not indicated.

Shaving, hair care, dental hygiene, upper and lower extremity dressing have improved and the patient is now independent. Minimal assistance is required for showering due to the patient's impulsive behavior and decreased awareness of safety hazards while in the shower. A left side neglect continues to be evident; however, it does not interfere in the performance of functional activities.

Mr. A. was trained in the use of various one-handed adaptive devices and techniques for cold and light meal preparation. With structure, he is able to perform the activity safely with familiar recipes. The anticipation of errors is moderately impaired with new recipes, and the patient's wife has been instructed in the process of structuring the task to eliminate errors. Meals on Wheels is no longer needed.

Initially, the patient demonstrated a flaccid left upper extremity. After an increase in range of motion thus resulting in a decrease in pain, the patient was found to have some active movement in the shoulder. The patient developed moderate edema in the left upper extremity, which at the time of discharge was under control through aggressive therapy. Instruction for home follow-up with an emphasis in positioning was given to the patient and wife. The patient is now able to use the left upper extremity as a gross stabilizer.

Although the patient was very motivated to improve, family support was questionable as there was poor follow-through. Significant problems with family dynamics were reported by the patient, and a referral was made to the psychosocial services department for family intervention.

The patient has progressed to a level in which a plateau has been reached due to the poor family support and the current living arrangement. It appears that once the family problems have been resolved, the patient may be appropriate for further skilled occupational therapy.

_____ OTR

The introduction should state the reason for referral, the date of the initial assessment report, and the total number and type of treatments received. The physical findings section should state the final status of the abnormal findings reported in your initial assessment report and summarize the critical incidents and goal achievement for each goal listed in the treatment plan.

The discharge plans section should summarize the equipment needed, home activities, patient education, caregiver training, and referral to outside agencies. The final activities assessment section should state the final functional level obtained and any assistance required to maintain this level. If additional care in another setting or at a future time could benefit the patient, say so. Conclude the discharge summary with the statement, "The patient is now discharged" and your signature.

Streamlining Documentation

Reporting requirements may seem unwieldy for occupational therapists with clinical responsibilities, yet they are no less important than providing the best clinical care. To meet the professional and industry standards for content and format of your reports, you will want to find ways to streamline this report writing process.

The three essential elements of an efficient report writing system are:

1. clinical protocols
2. standardized measures and data collection forms
3. automated database reporting system

The challenge facing all clinical managers is to coordinate measurement schemes, data collection, and retrieval forms into occupational therapy reports in an efficient and effective way.

Ask yourself, "What would I do if I had immediate access to all my clinical data in any form I wanted?" Before installing yet another unworkable system, computerized or not, take time to reflect on how you and your staff would benefit from automated reporting.

Computerization will give you legible notes, trackable progress statements, outcome data on similar patients, and ease in searching for and retrieving clinical information. Unfortunately, automation alone will not reduce your report writing time or improve the quality of your reports unless your data collection process is standardized. Establishing and following specific clinical protocols and using objective measures (e.g., range of motion measures and skill performance codes) will help you streamline this process. Figures 6.6 and 6.7 present two checklists for reviewing your documentation. The first recaptures the format headings that should be included in the three types of documents described above; the second lists specific content that should be included in your assessment report.

Once you have your protocols, measures, and forms standardized and in place, you will want to find ways to automate your reporting system and to facilitate the translation of information you collect into formal occupational therapy reports that serve to justify payment for your services. Remember that data collection forms are only tools; they must be transformed to communicate with a wider audience. Computer-assisted documentation software and advanced word processing packages can help you do this. Automated database reporting systems also offer you a decision-support system by giving you immediate information on expected outcomes, monitoring response to treatment, urging timely treatment modification, and predicting future functional status.

Figure 6.6 Format checklists for occupational therapy documents

Assessment Report	Treatment Plan	Progress Reports
❑ Introduction	❑ Problems	❑ Dates of treatment
❑ Physical findings	❑ Goals	❑ Treatments performed
❑ Selection of activities	❑ Specific interventions/ methods	❑ Patient response
❑ Interpretation of findings	❑ Frequency	❑ Goals achieved
	❑ Duration of treatment	❑ Limitations remaining
		❑ Treatment plan modifications

Listed below are some documentation and database software products that can help you. The companies and products included in this list have been selected from more than 750 potential sources. Each company listed has product information suggesting that the product will be useful in streamlining the documentation of occupational therapy services. You are encouraged to inquire about the services and products offered relevant to your needs. Neither the authors nor AOTA, however, endorses the companies or products listed.

Automated Charting Systems

CliniCom International. (619) 456-0361. Software that automates a complete medical record. May be purchased in modules; has narrative components, initial evaluation, and progress and discharge summaries.

Calyx Corporation. (800) 558-2208. User-designed medical records. Facility structures both type of data entry and report format.

Medical Accounts Group. (800) 444-6244. "Smart Chart" uses a modified Weed Problem-Oriented Medical Record format. Software maintains a database and generates a clinical report.

Database Reports

Computer Notes. (800) 227-6683. A computerized notewriting system using bar codes to access the database. This electronic dictation system aids daily note writing.

Swanson & Company. (213) 438-5799. GO Application Software generates reimbursement reports (e.g., Therapy Attachment) and includes decision-support and a user-defined report logic and format. Software creates a clinical database for quality assurance.

Program Evaluation Systems

Parkside Associates. (708) 698-9866. Develops and maintains in- and outpatient (LORS/LADS and ROPES) program evaluation

Figure 6.7 Content checklist for an occupational therapy assessment report

Check if specific items have been included in your occupational therapy assessment report.

Introduction

Evaluation date .... ❑
Name .... ❑
Age/Sex .... ❑
Referral source and date .... ❑
Referral purpose .... ❑
Medical diagnosis and onset date .... ❑
Treatment diagnosis and onset date .... ❑

History

Relevant medical history .... ❑
Relevant vocational history .... ❑
Relevant family history .... ❑
Previous functional level .... ❑
Socioeconomic status .... ❑
Educational status .... ❑
Residential status .... ❑
Current functional status .... ❑
Resource information .... ❑

Previous therapy received .... ❑
Concurrent therapy (if applicable) .... ❑

Physical findings

Summary of information .... ❑
   Initial interview regarding activity
     performance and services requested .... ❑
   Observation of patient's activity performance .... ❑

Interpretation of findings

Objective functional disabilities identified
   in functional activities .... ❑
Physical and cognitive assistance levels identified .... ❑
Response to assistance stated .... ❑
Need for assistive devices identified .... ❑
Adaptations or compensations needed identified .... ❑
Long-term goals identified .... ❑
Unusual precautions/contraindications stated .... ❑
Rehabilitation potential stated .... ❑

Treatment plan (may be separate document or included in assessment report by facility choice)

Treatment plan addresses stated problems .... ❑
Goals identified .... ❑
Specific methods stated .... ❑
Specific frequency and duration of treatment stated .... ❑

systems. Standardized measures generate program evaluation reports for comparison.

Marianjoy Rehabilitation Center. (312) 462-4202. Participating institutions submit functional assessments (PECS) and other patient information to the center. The center maintains a database for each institution and performs routine and ad hoc analyses.

Uniform Data Systems. (716) 831-2076. Managed by the Center for Functional Assessment Research, SUNY Buffalo. Subscribers use the Functional Independence measure and receive training and quarterly reports.

Easter Seal. (312) 667-7400. Provides rehabilitation management software; seven modules, including a CARF module. Includes report generation with editing capability.

References

American Medical Association. (1984). *Guides to the evaluation of permanent impairment* (2nd ed.). Chicago, IL: Author.

American Occupational Therapy Association. (1989). *Uniform terminology for occupational therapy* (2nd ed.). Rockville, MD: Author.

Medicare Hospital Manual Publication 10. (1968). Chapter IV, Washington, D.C.: Department of Health and Human Services, Health Care Financing Administration, 406-408.

Weed, L.L. (1971). *Medical records, medical education, and patient care: The problem-oriented record as a basic tool.* Chicago: Year Book.

7. A Payer's Review of Documentation

Claudia Allen, MA, OTR, FAOTA
Mary Foto, OTR, FAOTA
Terry Moon-Sperling, OTR
Dorothy Wilson, OTR, FAOTA

This chapter describes the medical review process necessary for Medicare claims. Although other third party payers may not require the technical detail or monthly certification that Medicare requires, the concepts and medical review process are applicable for all reimbursement sources. This article originally appeared in the December 1989 issue of the American Journal of Occupational Therapy *and is reprinted here with permission.*

Claudia Allen is an occupational therapy consultant, Blue Cross of California, Van Nuys, CA.

Mary Foto is a senior allied health consultant, Blue Cross of California, Van Nuys, CA.

Terry Moon-Sperling is an occupational therapy consultant, Blue Cross of California, Van Nuys, CA.

Dorothy Wilson is an occupational therapy consultant, Blue Cross of California, Van Nuys, CA.

After a patient has received occupational therapy services and the provider has sent the bill for services to the fiscal intermediary (an insurance company that contracts with the federal government to process Medicare claims), a medical review may take place to ensure that the services provided are covered under Medicare regulations. At the beginning of 1989, the Health Care Financing Administration (HCFA) introduced new guidelines for these occupational therapy reviews, called "Outpatient Occupational Therapy Medicare Part B Guidelines" (see boxed material on opposite page). These guidelines speed the process of reimbursement, yet also require that providers complete their Part B bills (UB-82 form) with 100% accuracy.

The purpose of this chapter is to explain the medical review process via a focus on occupational therapy claims and an outline of what medical reviewers must have before providers can be reimbursed for services. A documentation example that includes the elements to establish medical necessity is also provided.

The Importance of Proper Documentation

As Medicare medical reviewers for Blue Cross of California and practicing occupational therapists, we have an opportunity to observe the medical review process from both perspectives. We understand the problems involved when a claim is denied or sent back to the provider for further information, and we have found that thorough documentation is the key to successful reimbursement.

Documentation requirements may seem trivial when compared with the complex and, at times, overwhelming degrees of disabilities that patients present. However, responsibility for proper documentation of services is no less important than the selection of the most effective treatment approach or the provision of the best clinical care. Documentation is the only tangible evidence of the critical link between the therapist's clinical reasoning and the patient's functional performance outcome. Improper documentation can result in a claim being denied or returned to the provider for additional information, thus jeopardizing the patient's access to further treatment.

When a claim is denied for technical reasons, the billing office and the beneficiary receive a claims correction notice, which provides basic information concerning the denial. When the claim is denied for medical necessity, a Medicare denial letter is sent. The occupational therapist should review denied cases individually and determine if an additional technical requirements review or a medical necessity review is warranted.

Technical Requirements Review

The first step in a medical review for most fiscal intermediaries, including Blue Cross of California, is to screen specific areas of the claim or bill and to check that these areas are completed and that the information fulfills the requirements for an outpatient Part B bill. During this initial technical—or Level I—review, the areas typically checked are the ICD-9 diagnosis code (the diagnosis related to the occupational therapy treatment), the onset date for

A Provider's Guide to HCFA Rules and Medicare Interpretations

There is a difference between Health Care Financing Administration (HCFA) regulations, which are issued by HCFA in Baltimore, and interpretations of regulations, which are done by HCFA regional offices, the fiscal intermediaries, and their medical reviewers.

Regulations and guidelines are sent directly to providers by HCFA headquarters in Baltimore. An example is Health Insurance Manuals, which are general guidelines, distinguished by type of facility. Each Health Insurance Manual giving Part A and Part B information has three sections: one on general information, one on coverage of services, and one on billing procedures.

HCFA clarifies the Health Insurance Manual with transmittals. Four recent transmittals (1989), written to deal with a perceived lack of standards in Part B occupational therapy medical reviews, are (a) No. 281, for skilled nursing facilities; (b) No. 565, for acute care hospitals; (c) No. 223, for home health care; and (d) No. 87, for rehabilitation agencies and comprehensive outpatient rehabilitation facilities. These four transmittals contain similar information.

In addition to the Health Insurance Manual, HCFA publishes and updates a Coverage Issues Manual with details on selected topics across all disciplines. For example, the Cardiac Rehabilitation section of the Coverage Issues Manual (Reference No. 35-25) is updated every few years. Although the content changes, the reference number of the updates remains the same. The Coverage Issues Manual includes valuable information on the available benefits and exclusions of the Medicare program.

A fiscal intermediary is an insurance company that has a contract with the government to process Medicare Part A claims for payment. Each fiscal intermediary is assigned to one of nine HCFA regional offices. The HCFA central office provides direction and coordination responsibilities within the Social Security Administration for the Medicare program.

HCFA regulations establish the framework from which interpretations may be made. Each HCFA region provides additional structure to HCFA guidelines. Both the regional office and the fiscal intermediary use professional community standards to assist in the interpretation of regulations to meet the needs of the Medicare beneficiary. The medical reviewers are instrumental in monitoring both community standards and current interpretations of Medicare guidelines.

To keep the providers informed, each fiscal intermediary publishes Medicare bulletins and periodically holds workshops on billing and medical coverage issues. Blue Cross of California, for example, has published updates on a variety of issues, including certification, billing, and therapy guidelines. To obtain information on workshops and other services, the therapists should contact the fiscal intermediary that processes their Medicare claims.

the treatment diagnosis, the start-of-care date, the dates of service, the number of treatment visits for the period billed, and the total dollar amount for the treatment visits.

At Blue Cross of California, if all of these areas meet the requirements, the claim will pass the Level I review and be paid right away. If, however, these basic technical requirements are not met, the claim is reviewed for medical necessity (Level II review).

Clerical Errors

Many technical errors can be traced to improper coding for diagnosis and treatment; perhaps the billing clerk responsible for completing the claim has misunderstood an occupational therapist's notes or has had little experience in proper coding. Common errors at this level include the following:

- The diagnosis on the bill differs from the diagnosis of concern to the occupational therapist. For example, the diagnosis code on the bill may indicate that the diagnosis is urinary incontinence, but the diagnosis that caused the referral to the occupational therapist is cerebrovascular accident. It is essential to specify the diagnosis used to establish the occupational therapist's goals.
- The number of treatment units is mistaken for the number of visits, thereby causing the number of visits to appear excessive for the billing period.
- The start-of-care date and the onset date are the same. Except for an emergency room visit, the start-of-care date typically occurs after the onset date. For example, the date of the onset of multiple sclerosis would be prior to the date of the first day of therapy.

These clerical errors cause a delay in claim processing because additional or corrected information is required before the final review of the claim. The occupational therapist can reduce these delays by making sure that the billing office has accurate information. (Blue Cross of California provides a form for recording such information.)

Education to increase billing accuracy can be provided through workshops, printed materials, audiotapes, and computer programs. One such computer program, PT Medicode+, developed by Blue Cross of California (1989), addresses the billing problems specifically cited by the American Occupational Therapy Association ("Update on Medicare," 1988). Although originally designed to assist in physical therapy billing, this software program also pertains to occupational therapy billing and is available in two versions: 1500 for private practices and UB-82 for hospitals, rehabilitation facilities, nursing homes, and home health care agencies.

Request for Medical Records

When a claim falls outside the norms established by Level I review for the fiscal intermediary, the third party payer may request that the provider supply medical information for further investigation into the claim. This request does not indicate an automatic denial; it simply represents a reviewer's desire for further clarification to ensure a fair and objective decision on the case.

For a complete, fair, and accurate review, these medical records must include documentation of the following:

- the patient's medical history (supplied by a physician or through an interview with the therapist)
- a physician's referral
- physician certification
- an initial evaluation
- daily documentation from the start-of-care date
- weekly and monthly progress notes
- an itemized financial ledger showing daily charges

The third party payer's medical reviewer then uses the concurrent review form (see Figure 13.2 on page 150) to ascertain that technical requirements have been met and to determine if the therapy provided is at a covered level of care.

A request for medical records is initiated well after services have been provided. The following is a guideline for the provision of complete documentation of services and for the avoidance of deficient records.

Patient's Medical History
These records, which are supplied by the physician or through an interview with the therapist, should provide supportive information to substantiate the need for the stated intervention.

Physician's Referral
A physician's referral should include the following:

- the occupational therapy treatment diagnosis
- the onset date of the treatment diagnosis
- the actual or estimated date of any recent change in level of function
- a request for evaluation or specific orders
- the date and the physician's signature

If the physician has ordered an evaluation, the therapist should establish a treatment plan (including the type of activity or procedure and the frequency and duration of treatment) at the time of the initial evaluation and sign and date this plan. Any changes or additions to this plan should be in writing and should be signed and dated by the occupational therapist. If the physician has ordered a specific occupational therapy plan, the specific orders must be followed unless the therapist suggests or receives a change in orders from the physician. All telephone orders must be documented and then signed by the physician as required by state law and by facility and occupational therapy department procedures. Common errors in the physician's referral that cause delays or technical denials include incomplete or nonspecific orders (e.g., PRN orders), orders with a span of frequency and duration (e.g., two to three times a week for 4 to 6 weeks), and orders that do not state a specific type of treatment (e.g., activities as needed).

Physician Certification
Certification for outpatient services is a statement written by the physician at the time treatment is begun indicating that the patient needs occupational therapy services. This certification is good for 30 days from the date of the initial evaluation or the start-of-care date. Blue Cross of California accepts the initial physician's referral as the first certification. On or before the 30th day of treatment and every 30 days thereafter, recertification must be obtained in writing and signed and dated by the physician. The use of a stamp for the physician's signature on orders, certification, or recertification is not valid. The original certification and recertifications with the physician's signature should be kept on file.

Certification or recertification may be in any form, but must contain the following key elements:

- a statement that the physician has seen the patient during the 30-day period
- a statement of the need for continuing outpatient occupational therapy
- a statement estimating the length of time services will be needed to achieve the treatment goals
- a statement of the physician's intention to review the case every 30 days

Initial Evaluation

These records must contain baseline data—both subjective and objective—that measure the relevant recovery factors for that patient's treatment diagnosis. Goals must be clearly stated and must relate directly to the baseline recovery factors.

Daily Documentation from the Start-of-Care Date

At a minimum, daily documentation should state the date of treatment, type of treatment, length of the treatment session if the therapist billed by time and procedure, and patient's progress, including documentation of changes whenever they occur. If no changes are occurring, that fact should be documented.

Weekly and Monthly Progress Notes

Brief weekly notes stating changes from the beginning of the treatment week and monthly summaries of changes from the beginning of the treatment month are required. Changes in the patient's ability to perform activities of daily living from one period to the next are summarized.

In daily, weekly, and monthly notes, the therapist should measure and document changes in key factors previously identified as contributing to the patient's decreased function. Relevant factors, such as pain, loss of range of motion, loss of functional ability to follow or retain instruction, and attitude, are frequently related to the patient's performance. The notes should clearly state when the patient reaches a goal. Likewise, if the patient has not reached a goal, an explanation should be provided.

To demonstrate that adequate supervision has been given, the daily notes of all occupational therapy assistants and aides must be cosigned as required by state regulation and Medicare's conditions of participation.

Itemized Financial Ledger Showing Daily Charges

Itemized services that are billed on the financial ledger must match the daily occupational therapy treatment record. All services billed must be covered by benefits of the Medicare insurance program. Treatments such as biofeedback training for relaxation, driver's education, and case conferences are not covered by the program.

To avoid technical denials, we recommend that the occupational therapy department be responsible for reviewing the medical records before they are sent to the intermediary to ensure that they are clear and complete, include all items requested, and reflect the billing period in question. The therapist should include the complete records from the start-of-care date. Determination of the patient's progress for the billing period under review is difficult without the initial evaluation, treatment notes, and summaries from previous billing periods. The intermediary usually does not keep all of the previous medical records on file.

If a claim is questioned because technical requirements are not met, the areas concerning medical necessity are not reviewed. In the medical review process, the quality of a therapist's services may not matter if technical requirements have not been properly addressed. The denial of reimbursement because of technical problems is troubling to a clinician.

Medical Necessity Review

Medicare denies coverage for the following basic reasons:

1. *The need for the occupational therapist's unique skills and knowledge is not evident.* Covered treatment must be at a certain level of complexity and sophistication, or the condition of the patient must be such that the treatment can be performed safely and effectively only by a certified occupational therapist or under such a therapist's supervision. If the patient or caregiver could provide the care (e.g., activities of daily living routines, endurance activities, exercises, transfers) or if the treatment consists of instructions that another service could provide, then skilled occupational therapy is considered unnecessary.

2. *The patient would improve naturally without the help of an occupational therapist.* If the general progression of the patient's medical condition would return the patient to a previous level of functioning spontaneously, then skilled occupational therapy intervention is not considered to be medically necessary.

3. *The patient shows no significant improvement within a reasonable and predictable amount of time.* "Reasonable" is considered to mean that there is a greater than 50% probability that the patient will make significant improvement as a consequence of occupational therapy. "Predictable amount of time" is interpreted to mean that the planned frequency and duration of treatments is a knowledgeable estimate of how long it will take the patient to achieve therapy goals in relation to the diagnosis, severity, and prognosis of the condition. If at any point in the course of the treatment it is determined that the expectations will not materialize, occupational therapy services will no longer be considered reasonable. If treatment of underlying factors, such as an increase in endurance, strength, or range of motion, or a decrease in pain, does not improve the performance of functional activities, then improvement is not considered to be significant.

4. *The patient has not demonstrated sustainable gains, is considered to be at a maintenance level, and is not expected to show further improvement.* Therapists must document decreased levels of assistance or improved patient responses to assistance provided. Documentation of activity outcomes should be stated in measurable, objective terms.

5. *The occupational therapy services duplicate services provided by other therapists.* If a single discipline, such as physical therapy, occupational therapy, speech therapy, or nursing, could provide the care, only one discipline can bill the charges. For example, if the occupational therapy program provided upper extremity exercises and the physical therapy program provided lower extremity exercises and gait training, then only physical therapy would be covered because physical therapy could also provide upper extremity exercises. If the occupational therapy program included transfers, dressing, and upper extremity exercises and the physical therapy program provided only upper extremity exercises, then only the occupational therapy would be covered. Services are not considered duplicative in cases where both services involved have unique treatment goals that lead to distinct functional outcomes. For example, in *transfer training*, the physical therapy goal is for safe and independent transfers, and the occupational therapy goal is for the appropriate use of transfer techniques in activities of daily living. In *brain injury rehabilitation*, the occupational therapy goal is to employ neuromuscular therapies to increase functional use of the upper extremity in dressing or bathing, and the physical therapy goal is to use neuromuscular therapies to assist the patient in the use of the upper extremity during ambulation activities.

Determining Medical Necessity

To determine medical necessity, the intermediary reviews the patient's medical records from the start-of-care date. In this review, the intermediary asks: Why does this patient need an occupational therapist now? The therapist's knowledge of disability and activity analysis must be combined with a reasonable expectation for improving functional performance.

The medical reviewer's role is to determine medical necessity on the basis of documentation in the medical records indicating that the patient's condition and level of function required the special knowledge and skill of an occupational therapist. As practicing therapists we focus on the patient's disability, but as medical reviewers we focus on whether the nature of that disability requires a therapist's knowledge to successfully help the patient.

Establishing Reasonability and Necessity of Services

To be covered by the fiscal intermediary, occupational therapy services must be reasonable and necessary. Services are "reasonable" if the patient has a fair or good rehabilitation potential for the established goals. A good rehabilitation potential exists when the patient's function is expected to improve significantly within a limited and predictable amount of time on the basis of the occupational therapist's initial assessment. Services are "necessary" if skilled occupational therapy is required to produce the expected improvement. If the expected improvement is not achieved, the intervening variables that invalidated the therapist's prediction of rehabilitation potential should be identified.

Documentation of the presence of a disability alone, however, is not enough. Therapists must identify the specific diagnosis (ICD-9 code) that substantiates the need for a skilled occupational therapist's assessment and must prove that the patient could only improve through the application of the therapist's special knowledge of activity analysis and treatment methods.

Documenting Treatment

To document treatment so that the medical reviewer does not need to search for treatment goals and for the patient's progress toward those goals, the therapist can use the following four steps as guidelines:

Step 1: The Initial Evaluation
In this step, the therapist asks, "Where are we?" and determines the patient's current levels through an initial evaluation. The initial evaluation begins with an interview of the patient, which is a crucial component of the evaluation and a prerequisite to the establishment of a practical treatment plan. The interview follows a complete review of the medical record and focuses on the perspective of the patient, the caregiver, or both. The interview establishes what activities the patient can perform, how often these activities are performed, and if the patient or caregiver is satisfied or dissatisfied with his or her performance. A successful interview uncovers the patient's perceived problems, physical or cognitive disabilities, relevant medical history, and available family and community support. The interview establishes a request for services by identifying areas in which the patient is doing well or poorly, and by screening out activities that are not relevant.

After the initial evaluation, a list of activities requested by the patient or caregiver is developed and improved upon with the special knowledge and skills of an occupational therapist. The therapist should document the patient's current levels for each of the requested activities. This is the starting point for the rest of the documentation.

Step 2: Rehabilitation Potential
In this step, the therapist asks, "Where are we going?" and "What are the specific, expected levels of activity for the patient?" The therapist then establishes measurable, realistic goals for the patient. Once the specific activities that can be improved through the intervention of an occupational therapist have been developed and the patient's current activity levels have been documented, the occupational therapist can determine the patient's expected levels. The therapist should write these expected levels as goals for each activity. Such goals must be measurable and must realistically

reflect the patient's rehabilitation potential. Each of these goals must be specifically relevant to the performance of functional activities. Ascertaining the patient's potential for improving functional status is a critical assessment decision for the therapist. It not only determines the type of therapy intervention that may be used but also enables the therapist to predict the outcome of the intervention on the patient's task performance.

Step 3: The Treatment Plan

In this step, the therapist asks, "How do we get there?" and "What specific treatments will bring the patient to the expected levels?" The therapist determines a specific treatment plan for each expected level identified in Step 2 and states the specific treatment plan and any changes in either the plan or its implementation. Documentation should include a record of treatment activities, modalities, and procedures; the patient's and family's education; the equipment ordered; the need for further evaluation; conferences with others; and discharge plans. The specifics of the discharge plan should be stated—that is, the amount of supervision required, the education of the patient and family that has been accomplished and that is still required, and a tentative discharge date.

Step 4: Assessment of the Patient's Progress

In this step, the therapist asks, "How are we doing?" The patient's progress is measured. This is the proof that the plan is working, the facts that prove that an occupational therapist is essential to the patient's progress. Each treatment diagnosis has a probable set of outcome alternatives. Once the treatment goal has been established, each progress note must reestablish the appropriateness of these goals and monitor the specific change the patient has made toward the goal.

Progress notes must contain a series of established causes and must measure progress and monitor functional outcome. Each note must reflect progress toward the determined goal. For example, if full range of motion of the shoulder is the goal, then the therapist should do the following:

- establish that the causative factor (pain) is being controlled
- measure the shoulder's passive, active, and functional range of motion
- monitor changes in specific tasks, for example, upper extremity dressing

Alternatively, the therapist could do the following:

- establish that muscle weakness is the underlying cause of shoulder immobility
- measure quantitative changes in strength
- monitor changes in specific tasks (e.g., independence in meal preparation at home)

By establishing causes and measuring progress, the therapist clearly outlines each step toward predetermined goals. This

Documentation Steps	Commonly Used Information (Insufficient)	Specific Information (Sufficient)
Step 1: Initial evaluation	Patient requires assistance with self-care.	The patient requires moderate physical assistance and step-by-step verbal cuing to dress (secondary to left-side neglect, decreased left upper extremity function, and diminished motor planning). The caregiver is not knowledgeable of compensatory dressing techniques and typically performs these tasks for patient.
Step 2: Rehabilitation potential	Instruct the patient in self-care.	The patient will achieve at least a minimum assistance level for dressing with the use of compensatory techniques. The caregiver will learn the proper methods and cues for assisting the patient.
Step 3: Treatment plan	Provide functional activities.	The therapist will provide dressing training and practice with the use of various compensatory techniques to determine the most suitable technique for the patient, combined with instruction of the caregiver to follow through.
Step 4: Assessment of the patient's progress	Patient improved in self-care.	The patient performs dressing with minimum assistance, requiring cuing for left arm placement into sleeve. The caregiver is able to demonstrate appropriate methods of assisting the patient.

method will help substantiate that the services of an occupational therapist are indeed necessary to secure reimbursement, thus allowing for further treatment for the patient. See Table 7.1 for an example of sufficient and insufficient documentation.

Conclusion   When reimbursement is denied or delayed, it is often due to insufficient documentation—either the documentation lacks technical accuracy or lacks details supporting medical necessity. We recommend that the therapist pay attention to the areas that are screened for accuracy and take the time to review claims before they are sent to the fiscal intermediary. Regardless of the fiscal intermediary or medical reviewer, however, the suggestions in this paper were made to assist occupational therapists in submitting complete documentation for outpatient Medicare reimbursement.

Because clerical errors cause the majority of technical errors, we suggest that billing clerks as well as therapists and administrators become familiar with claims coding. PT Medicode+, a software program designed specifically to decrease billing errors, may be useful in this endeavor.

The guidelines presented in this paper to help therapists keep medical records can be used to provide the information necessary for a fair review. By following these guidelines from the beginning of treatment, therapists will have proper documentation when records are requested. Additionally, the four steps of documentation that we provided should help therapists develop a clear image of a patient's progress and should substantiate the need for the specific skills of an occupational therapist, thus helping to establish medical necessity.

References

Blue Cross of California. (1989). PT Medicode+ [Computer program]. Van Nuys, CA: Author.

Health Care Financing Administration. *Coverage issues manual* (DHHS Publication No. 33-25). Baltimore, MD: Author.

Health Care Financing Administration. (1989). Outpatient occupational therapy Medicare part B guidelines (DHHS Transmittal No. 565). In *Health insurance manual*. Baltimore, MD: Author.

Update on Medicare denial appeals procedures. (1988, September). *Occupational Therapy News*, p. 8.

8. Writing Functional Goals

Patricia Mahoney, OTR/L
Kathleen Kannenberg, MA, OTR/L

Therapists frequently say that writing good functional goals is the most difficult aspect of documentation. We have also learned that goal setting will guide the direction of subsequent note writing. Perhaps that explains why the majority of reimbursement problems occur because of poor documentation. Therefore, if the goals are wrong, unclear, or incomplete, the entire set of notes may not paint a clear picture of the patient's functional status before and after treatment.

Patricia Mahoney is a case manager at New England Rehabilitation Hospital, Woburn, MA.

Kathleen Kannenberg is the mental health program manager for the American Occupational Therapy Association.

Increasing costs of health care have forced third party payers to look closely at what services they are paying for. The Health Care Financing Administration (HCFA) established The Medicare Part B guidelines in 1989 in order to clarify what services occupational therapists can expect to be reimbursed for under Medicare Part B in the outpatient setting. Because the Medicare Part B guidelines are the only thorough documentation guidelines in print, other insurers are beginning to adopt them when looking at reimbursement for services.

Medicare is not the only payer looking closely at documentation when deciding which services to reimburse. Commercial insurers are also paying more attention to how their dollars are spent. Often a commercial insurer will either have its own internal utilization review department or contract with a utilization review company or private case manager in order to monitor a patient's progress and make decisions regarding reimbursement. The health maintenance organizations (HMOs) will frequently conduct on-site reviews in hospitals and request documentation concurrently in outpatient settings.

All of the third party payers are looking for the same thing in terms of patient progress: changes in function. Reviewers are looking for documentation that indicates the patient is progressing, as evidenced by favorable functional outcomes. Occupational therapists need to document goals and progress toward goals in a functional manner that can be understood by the third party reviewer.

Occupational therapists need to document the underlying factors, e.g., range of motion (ROM), sensation, tone, and attention span, but they also need to link these factors to function. This process helps to focus the patient's treatment, as the functional outcome becomes more significant than any specific deficit the patient may have. For example, documenting increases in shoulder ROM is not helpful unless it is documented that the person has gained the ability to bathe independently as a result of the increased range. In the psychiatric occupational therapy setting, stating that a person is less depressed does not denote a change in function; however, documenting that the person can now dress with minimal cuing does demonstrate progress toward a functional goal.

Establishing Goals

The easiest way to accomplish writing a treatment plan that addresses function is to establish functional long-term and short-term goals. The Medicare B guidelines require that goals must be functional, measurable, and objective. In order for a goal to be functional, it must include a functional component, e.g., self-care, meal preparation, family teaching, social interaction, etc.

A goal is measurable and objective if it states the person's achievement in a way to make a goal measurable. The Medicare B guidelines include the levels of assistance that can be used to describe the person's progress. The levels of assistance described in the guidelines are helpful in that they include both the physical and cognitive levels. Using these levels of assistance helps to justify treating a person who may not have physical problems, but whose cognitive problems interfere with functioning in everyday life.

When writing functional goals, the therapist needs to document the functional level the patient is expected to achieve (e.g., "Patient will bathe lower body with minimal assist," or "Patient will make one purchase from the gift shop with moderate assist"). You also need to include the expected outcomes from the limiting factors when applicable, (e.g. "Patient will demonstrate 90° of shoulder flexion in order to don shirt independently," or "Patient will attend to cooking task for 20 minutes in order to prepare light meal with standby assist").

Traditionally, when occupational therapists begin evaluating patients, they look at the underlying factors first, e.g., ROM, strength, sensation, perception, cognition, etc. However, documenting functional levels first and then evaluating the limiting factors that affect the person's ability to complete functional activities will serve two purposes. First, there is no need to spend treatment time on particular underlying factors if they have no functional impact. For example, a patient may have limited shoulder ROM but still be able to do all self-care independently. Third party payers may not reimburse for treatment of a patient who has no functional deficit.

Secondly, by assessing functional activities/abilities first, it is easier to see where problems related to underlying factors interfere with function. For example, by assessing a person during bathing and dressing, it is possible to look at several areas of cognition and perception, such as sequencing, organization, memory, orientation, depth perception, apraxia, etc. The next step would be to look more closely at the areas where impairments are evident and conduct an in-depth evaluation.

In the same way, after evaluating a patient and finding that he or she needs maximum assist to perform hygiene tasks, it is then necessary to evaluate ROM, strength, communication, or other factors that limit the person's ability to function. This information assists in writing functional goals that are realistic and measurable (e.g., "Patient will demonstrate appropriate energy conservation techniques in order to independently prepare a light snack").

It may be helpful to structure the occupational therapy initial evaluation so that functional activities are placed first on the form. This will serve as a reminder to therapists to assess these areas first and then evaluate the underlying factors.

At times it may be difficult to relate a goal to a functional activity. It may be helpful to ask the patient what his or her prior functional level was, or what he or she cannot do that could be accomplished before the illness or injury.

It is also important to ask the patient and/or caregiver what his or her goals are. If the patient's goals are realistic, agreement between patient and therapist can be documented. If the patient's goals are unrealistic, the therapist gains valuable information for treatment planning.

It may be difficult at times to establish functional goals for patients who function at a higher level, e.g., independent with self-care, but unable to live independently. Goals addressing community skills or safety issues may be appropriate in this case. Referring to a checklist of activities may be helpful in establishing functional goals.

This list may include such activities as dialing 911 in an emergency, preparing menus, grocery shopping, handling money, balancing a checkbook, writing checks, doing laundry, arranging transportation for appointments, etc. Consider activities where safety is a factor. The generation of such an extensive list of functional activities should assist with establishing goals for patients at all levels.

The Treatment Plan

After evaluating the patient and discussing the patient's goals, the next step is to determine the treatment plan. The treatment plan includes both long-term and short-term goals. Long-term goals are written with the intent that they will be achieved at the time of discharge from therapy. Short-term goals are intended to be accomplished within the time frame of the long-term goals. Time frames can range anywhere from 1 week to 1 month or more. It is best to write short-term goals that are functional, keeping in mind that every short-term goal must be associated with a long-term goal.

If the long-term goal states that the patient will be able to shop independently for necessary grocery items, the short-term goal might be that the patient will be able to generate a shopping list with minimal assist. In this example, it is necessary to achieve the short-term goal prior to achieving the long-term goal of independence with grocery shopping.

Functional goals need to be written to show what the patient will accomplish, not what the therapist will do. Goals such as "Evaluate for cognitive deficits" or "Teach family car transfers" are part of the therapist's plan, not the patient's goals. If each goal is documented so that it starts with "Patient will…" or "Patient's family will…," all of the goals will be patient or caregiver goals.

Examples of Functional Goals

Functional goals might be written in the form shown in the following examples:

1. Patient will perform safe transfers on and off the toilet with standby assistance.
2. Patient will independently create a grocery store list from menus she has prepared.
3. Patient will demonstrate independence with home exercise program.
4. Patient's daughter will independently transfer patient into and out of the car from the wheelchair.
5. Patient will take a timeout when angry with peers in order to complete a group school assignment.

When the focus of treatment is one of the underlying factors, it is important to include these in the functional goals. Examples might include the following:

1. Patient will sustain attention to task for 10 minutes in order to prepare a light snack with standby assistance.
2. Patient will maintain eye contact when greeting visitors at the volunteer desk independently.
3. Patient will demonstrate 90° shoulder flexion in order to bathe back independently using equipment.
4. Patient will demonstrate right wrist extension of 10° in order to operate cash register independently.
5. Patient will use memory log book with minimal assist in order to follow a daily schedule.
6. Patient's family will demonstrate independence in positioning techniques so that the patient may eat with standby assistance.
7. Patient will use good body mechanics in order to vacuum independently.
8. Patient will be able to assertively express work concerns to supervisor with minimal assistance.

Although not every goal needs to include the underlying factors, it is important to identify the underlying factors that interfere with function. If the underlying factors are not addressed in the goal, they need to be addressed in the progress notes. For example, if the long-term goal is independent lower-extremity dressing, and decreased strength interferes with goal achievement, then progress in strength needs to be documented in the notes. Progress notes can be streamlined a great deal if documentation focuses on the functional problems and underlying factors. Goal achievement will address the functional gains. Objective data in the note may address progress with the underlying factors. The assessment should pull the progress note together by stating how gains in specific areas have increased overall function.

Identifying the functional problem and the underlying factors that contribute to the problem assists the treatment planning process. In this way, it becomes clear which areas need to be addressed and how progress will affect function. Patients remain in treatment until goals are achieved or the patient no longer makes progress. It is easier to identify patients who are ready for discharge when goals are written as functional outcomes. Patients are then discharged appropriately when goals are achieved.

Functional goals are appropriate for all treatment settings and any patient requiring occupational therapy services. This includes inpatient acute care and rehabilitation, outpatient facilities, work hardening programs, skilled nursing facilities, school systems, day-treatment programs, mental health facilities, and home health care. It may be difficult at first to establish functional goals for all patients, but this process becomes easier with practice.

Although not all third party payers are requiring that goals be functional, more and more reviewers of documentation are looking for functional progress and functional outcomes. In order to justify the need for occupational therapy services and ensure payment, all therapists need to look at their documentation with a critical eye and ask themselves, "Are these services necessary, and would I pay for these services?"

If therapists write goals that are functional, measurable, and objective, it will help to ensure that the answer to this question is yes.

9. Special Considerations I: Pediatrics

Barbara Chandler, MOT, OTR

In certain areas or settings of practice, there are special considerations that should be highlighted for the purposes of documentation. The areas of pediatrics, home health, and mental health have been selected because they are the most common areas causing difficulties. This chapter focuses on pediatrics, while chapters 10 and 11 deal with home health and mental health, respectively.

Barbara Chandler is the pediatric program manager for the American Occupational Therapy Association.

Documentation for occupational therapy services to pediatric clients shares many similarities with documentation of occupational therapy services for any client. Many of the suggestions for appropriate documentation stated elsewhere in this book are applicable and necessary for documentation for services to pediatric clients. Technical information such as name and insurance number must be correct. The documentation must be organized so that relevant information can be easily located. The services provided must have been skilled services provided by an occupational therapist to increase function. The services must also have been medically necessary. The notes of what occurred during treatment sessions must relate to the goals of the treatment plan. The service should not be a duplication of other services, although clear coordination of efforts with other services is desirable. The documentation must indicate, with some minor exceptions discussed later, steady progression from a dependent to a less dependent or, hopefully, an independent state.

There are, however, some important differences to consider when documenting some services for pediatric clients. In general, these differences cluster around two main topics: developmental considerations and educational considerations or relevance.

Developmental Considerations

Many occupational therapists have had experience with submitting claims to third party payers and being informed that the insurance policies did not cover any condition or disability that was developmental in nature. This is a particularly chilling revelation when one considers the vast needs of many children whose functional disabilities are identified early and who could clearly benefit from intervention and require far fewer and less extensive services, if any, later in life.

It may be helpful for occupational therapists treating children with developmental disabilities to clarify certain points in the documentation process. The difference between the primary medical diagnosis and the secondary treatment diagnosis must be clear. Occupational therapists do not treat medical diagnoses. Occupational therapists treat the secondary diagnosis or functional disabilities that result from the condition identified in the primary diagnosis.

For example, although occupational therapists treat many children with cerebral palsy, occupational therapists do not treat the cerebral palsy. Occupational therapists address the functional disabilities that result from the condition. Occupational therapists treat functional disabilities such as inability to feed oneself due to poor manipulation of eating utensils, or inability to dress oneself independently. Occupational therapists may treat the functional disability of poor sequencing skill resulting from seizure activity. Occupational therapists do not treat the seizures. Occupational therapists providing services to children with developmental disabilities must document the functional disabilities rather than the delay in the acquisition of developmental skills.

While age must be considered when setting goals and documenting, it is best not to describe the disability in age terms. One should not say that a child is 2 years behind in dressing skill, or write a goal that says to increase dressing skills to an age-appropriate level. One should write the goal in functional terms: Increase ability to dress oneself to an independent level. While this would be an appropriate goal for a 5-year-old, it would not be an appropriate goal for a 2-year-old despite the fact that the developmental delay suggests that this will be a functional disability in the future. A 2-year-old would not be expected to dress independently. A clear indication of progression from a dependent state to a less dependent or independent state should be evident in the documentation. Given the nature of developmental delays or disabilities, it is advisable to break the goals down into small enough increments so that progress can be clearly indicated within a reasonable time, usually a month.

Sensory Integration

Sensory integrative dysfunction or deficit may be considered a developmental disability by some third party payers or may be considered a condition that is not covered by certain policies or payers. Other payers may say sensory integrative treatment is an educationally related treatment approach. It is important when documenting the treatment provided to children with sensory integrative impairments that the treatment be identified as occupational therapy and that the functional disabilities resulting from the integrative problems be identified and described. Avoiding sensory integrative or developmental terms is advisable. The documentation should describe what the individual cannot do as a result of the integrative problems. The purpose of documentation is to communicate, and the majority of individuals reading the documentation, from parents to medical reviewers, are not going to be familiar with the neurological terms that are so familiar and clear to occupational therapists.

The developmental considerations can be summarized in on one word: *function*. Occupational therapists treat functional disabilities. The treatment diagnosis, the intervention goals, and the documentation of service provision must all address functional disabilities and functional goals. If function is the core of the documentation process, it is clearly communicated to anyone who reads the documentation. If function is expressed in terms of moving a child along a continuum from dependence to independence, the question of developmental delay is less likely to arise.

Educational Relevance

The second major consideration in pediatric documentation and one that is becoming increasingly complex is the issue of educational relevance for occupational therapy services provided in the public schools through an Individualized Education Program (IEP) under Part A of the Individuals with Disabilities Education Act (formerly the Education of the Handicapped Act). In Part A, occupational therapy is defined as a related service to special education. Related services are defined as "...transportation, and such developmental, corrective, and other supportive services as are required to assist a handicapped child to benefit from special education,..." (Code of Federal Regulations, 34, §300.13). Since a related service is tied to the need for special education, it is imperative that the occupational therapy intervention be clearly linked to the goals and objectives contained in the current IEP because it is the IEP that delineates what the special education will consist of and what services the child will receive.

Individualized Educational Program

Many occupational therapists have experienced difficulty in clearly explaining to special educators and other members of an IEP committee how disability and intervention needs identified by the occupational therapist are tied to educational goals and objectives. Often the "OT IEP section" along with the "speech IEP section" and the "adaptive PE IEP section", for example, are all stapled to the back of the educational IEP and presented to the parents as a comprehensive IEP. This is not how an IEP should be developed, and it contributes to the difficulty in explaining how occupational therapy is needed for the child to benefit from special education.

An IEP is developed by an IEP team (whose core members are identified in the Code of Federal Regulations, 34, §300.344). If the occupational therapy evaluation indicates that the child has deficits that interfere with educational functioning, the occupational therapist should attend the IEP meeting and contribute to the development of team consensus goals and objectives. The team consensus goals and objectives may require the services of more than one professional and should reflect the overall needs of the student.

For example, the team consensus goal of increased oral participation in class may require the input of the classroom teacher for management of a language group activity, the input of the speech pathologist to determine the grammatical area that will be focused on, and the input of the occupational therapist to determine a good postural position to enable the student to do the task. No one professional is going to be able to address this goal and the student's need alone. The occupational therapist may still address areas traditionally thought of as "OT," but always tie them to the educational (consensus) goal of increased oral participation in class. When an IEP is written and implemented in this way, the link between therapeutic goals and objectives and educational goals and objectives is clear.

Occupational therapists providing services in the schools should follow the same general guidelines for documentation as occupational therapists practicing in other settings. A detailed discussion of documenting occupational therapy services in school systems is available in the publication *Guidelines to Occupational Therapy Services in School Systems, Second Edition* (American Occupational Therapy Association, 1989).

Payment for Services in the Schools

Many school districts are now accessing third party payers for related services that are provided as part of a student's IEP. Since the related service must be educationally necessary and the reimburser covers services that are medically necessary, many questions have arisen about the overlap between these two types of services and the need for documentation that would satisfy the requirements of both the educational and medical systems. School system caseloads, ethics, and common sense dictate that it is impractical to have two sets of documentation for the same service. This apparent dilemma is easily resolved once practitioners providing services in the schools develop their goals and objectives in conjunction with the other members of the IEP committee and focus their goals, objectives, and documentation on functional disabilities and functional outcomes.

It should be noted that there may be services that are educationally necessary but not medically necessary and vice versa. No goals can be said to be clearly educational or clearly medical without considering the context of the child's individual situation. Each decision of medical and/or educational relevance must be based on the child's needs. Occupational therapy services in the schools are based on the individual needs of the child, and the decision on whether or how to provide occupational therapy services to a child eligible for special education should never be determined by the availability of a third party to pay for the service. The Individuals with Disabilities Education Act (formerly EHA) also clearly states that services are to be provided to students who need the service to benefit from special education. Unlike provisions required by third party payers, there is no requirement that students show progress in order to continue to receive occupational therapy in the school system.

Functional Disability

It is important to identify a functional disability and determine a functional goal or objective to address that disability. Documentation should be organized to reflect the relationship between the functional disability and the goal or objective to address that functional disability. The functional disability may be reflected (though not actually described) in the current level of educational functioning, which is a key component of the IEP. The wording of current level of educational functioning should be stated positively, e.g., "Reads four words;" "Identifies six letters of the alphabet;" or "Writes first letter of name." It should not be stated in terms of the functional disability, e.g., "Doesn't read at grade level;" "Doesn't identify 20 letters of the alphabet;" or "Doesn't write first name."

A comparison between current level of educational functioning and expected level of educational functioning for age and grade level will indicate educational deficit areas. If the occupational therapist can clearly see a link between the functional disabilities identified through the occupational therapy evaluation and the educational deficits, occupational therapy is appropriate as a related service.

The occupational therapist would indicate on the IEP how the remediation of the functional disabilities (stated as functional goals) would contribute to the educational goal. This is done by including the functional goals as intermediate steps (short-term objectives) toward the annual educational goal. Although the occupational therapist may work on many component parts of the functional goal, the component parts are never identified as the educational goal on the IEP. They are addressed as components and are only included in the therapeutic process because their remediation or improvement contributes to the functional goal (which in turn contributes to the attainment of the educational goal). In some instances, the functional goal and the educational goal may be the same.

The following three examples of parts of this process may help to illustrate these points.

Example 1
Tim is a 6-year-old student enrolled in a regular kindergarten. He is identified as a special needs student who has an orthopedic disability. He is currently dependent in all aspects of self-care and is unable to use any writing instrument. He maneuvers his wheelchair in the school building (level surface) at the rate of 1 foot per minute.

Appropriate educational goals for Tim may include the following:

1. Increase, to minimal assistance level, the ability to use the toilet.
2. Increase ability to manipulate objects to assist in performing daily living activities, e.g., dressing, eating, toileting, and writing.
3. Increase, to independent level, ability to maneuver wheelchair in the school building.
4. Increase self-feeding ability to an independent level.

These goals developed by the IEP team, including the occupational therapist, are educational because they address issues that:

1. Tim needs to be able to do to function independently in a classroom and during the school day.
2. Allow Tim to be served in the least restrictive environment, which is a primary goal of special education.
3. Require less adult supervision or assistance and would promote social interaction with Tim's peers since he would be participating in the same activities in similar, if not the same, ways as his peers.
4. Indicate progression on the road to independent adult functioning, which is the goal of public education in general.

All of the above goals are also written in functional terms that would satisfy the requirements of a third party payer.

The actual occupational therapy intervention may consist of activities that address the components or underlying impairments that interfere with the attainment of the functional goal. For example, Tim may need to improve his balance, grip strength, and oral-motor skills before he can feed himself independently. However, documentation of therapy sessions that addressed these component parts would always tie them to the functional goal of self-feeding. Poor mobility and balance, decreased endurance, difficulty sequencing, and inability to manipulate closures may all interfere with the ability to toilet independently. These component parts are appropriate to address in therapeutic intervention, but the intervention notes should always tie the component to the functional goal of more independent toileting.

A common educational goal is to improve handwriting. Although it is included in goal 2, it may also appear on the IEP as a separate annual goal. The therapist may address this by stating it functionally in terms of manipulating objects to perform daily living activities. Zippers, snaps, toys, pencils, utensils, tools, and telephones are all objects that may need to be manipulated in the home, school, or community. The occupational therapist may need to address muscle tone, grip, tactile perception, and visual-spatial skills to assist Tim in reaching this goal, but the intervention documentation would always link the activities to the functional goal of activity performance, e.g., eating, writing, etc.

Tim needs to be able to move his wheelchair in the school building to get from class to the library, cafeteria, bus area, etc. The occupational therapist may need to address poor sustained grip, low endurance, bilateral coordination, and visual-spatial orientation to assist Tim in improving his ability to move around the school in a timely and independent manner. Documentation of the occupational therapy intervention would always tie the treatment interventions and environmental modifications to the functional goal of independent mobility.

Example 2
A child with a learning disability may show tactile defensiveness with high activity level, distractibility, and poor motor planning. The therapeutic functional goal written to demonstrate educational relevance may read as follows:

- Increase ability to attend to multiple-step directions to carry out daily activities and learn new skills or compensatory techniques.

That kind of skill is clearly needed in the educational environment and is also a reimbursable functional goal. The skill is needed to learn new tasks, to sequence activities appropriately, to have adequate safety awareness and response, and to participate in social relationships.

The occupational therapist may address the tactile defensiveness as a contributing factor to the poor ability to attend to multiple-step directions, but the intervention documentation should clearly link the intervention focus to the functional goal.

Example 3

The special education for an older student may need to focus on prevocational or transition activities. Occupational therapy treatment plans that focus on the functional abilities (for example, appropriate work habits or behaviors) that are prevocational in nature and can be generalized to many situations, will usually be covered by third party payers; they are educationally relevant if there is an annual goal in the IEP or ITP (Individual Transition Plan) that focuses on work habits or behaviors. Supported employment programs, which may be a part of transition programs in the schools, usually focus on vocational skills and are unlikely to be considered medically necessary and, thus, reimbursable.

Linking the occupational therapy intervention to functional goals that contribute to the attainment of educational goals will solve both the problem of articulating how occupational therapy services are related to educational progress and will satisfy the requirements of a third party payer if one is involved with service provision in the school system.

Summary

The key to effective documentation in pediatrics is the key to effective documentation in all aspects of occupational therapy. The key is to address function.

References

American Occupational Therapy Association. (1989). *Guidelines for occupational therapy services in school systems* (2nd ed.). Rockville, MD: Author.

Chandler, B.E. (1989). Fee for service in the public schools. In *Program guide: The AOTA practice symposium* (pp. 34-37). Rockville, MD: American Occupational Therapy Association.

Code of Federal Regulations, 34, parts 300 to 399. (1990). Washington, DC: U.S. Government Printing Office.

10. Special Considerations II: Home Health

Velma Reichenbach, MS, OTR/L

This chapter, like the previous one, highlights special considerations affecting a certain area of practice. In this case, the author discusses special considerations affecting documentation in home health.

Velma Reichenbach is the supervisor of acute occupational therapy services, Mercy Hospital, Chicago, IL.

The demands on occupational therapists for documentation of service continues to challenge those providing therapy in the home health setting. In order to ensure reimbursement, the documentation must adhere to the rules established by service providers, government agencies, and accreditation organizations while also proving the necessity and uniqueness of occupational therapy as a skilled health care service.

Occupational therapy in home health is an exciting adventure because each patient shows functional performance deficits for a wide variety of reasons. The therapist's role is to search out the sensorimotor, cultural/psychosocial, cognitive, and perceptual dysfunctions that affect the patient's ability to perform. This information is elicited in each treatment session, and the puzzle is gradually documented as hypotheses are made and refined during the treatment.

The occupational therapist continues to observe the smallest details and provide the patient with the elements to elicit hope and make progress. Every treatment is an ongoing observation session, and the investigation continually leads to new goals. Hypotheses are switched or elaborated upon; goals are changed, enhanced, or deleted. In home health this is superlatively done—juggling the patient's sensorimotor, psychosocial/cultural, cognitive, and perceptual deficits with treatment goals, family dynamics, and architectural barriers. Indeed nowhere in occupational therapy practice is there such an opportunity to use a "holistic" approach incorporating a variety of occupational therapy theories.

Even the most experienced and rounded therapist may find documentation a drudgery. However, it is the avenue through which we demonstrate the importance and value of occupational therapy. If documentation is looked upon as the ingredient that allows us to provide needed service and promotion of the profession, it not only becomes tolerable, but also challenging and enjoyable. A picture of the patient is painted at the same time that what we do, how we do it, and our anticipated hopes for the patient's future are presented.

One recent article states, "Improper documentation can result in a claim being denied or returned to the provider for additional information thus jeopardizing the patient's access to further treatment" (Allen, Foto, Moon-Sperling, & Wilson, 1989, p. 783). Another source states the following related to the philosophy of documentation, "Every plan of treatment (claim) submitted to an intermediary represents an opportunity to educate a third-party payer. Every plan of treatment written and submitted to a third-party agency is an act of patient advocacy. The quality of our documentation is a measure of our professional credibility. Clear and accurate documentation reflects sound clinical reasoning" (Gillard & Kern, 1991).

Documentation Must Reflect Reimbursement Parameters

Under Medicare, the patient must be confined to his or her home, under the care of a physician, and in need of skilled nursing services, physical, or speech therapy on an intermittent basis.

Coverage under Medicare for home health benefits is reimbursable under both Parts A and B. The need for occupational therapy alone does not qualify a patient for the home health benefit. One of the other services must be required before occupational therapy can be introduced. However, occupational therapy may continue after the other skilled services have discharged the patient. One visit by a nurse to open the case does not constitute "intermittent." However, one visit required of the nurse in a 60-day period would constitute "intermittent."

The patient must be homebound or confined to his or her home. This means that to leave home requires considerable effort or taxing effort and the assistance of another person. Physician appointments are permitted, and an occasional trip to the barber shop might not be questioned. Denials do occur based upon the questioning of homebound status. Care must be taken to provide ongoing documentation indicating the patient is confined to the home.

Other requirements that apply include the following:

- The treatment requires a prescription.
- The treatment must be performed by a qualified occupational therapist or occupational therapy assistant.
- Treatment must be reasonable and necessary.
- Treatment must result in significant practical improvement in functioning in a predictable amount of time based on diagnosis, severity, and prognosis.
- Valid expectation of improvement must exist at the time of assessment although the expectation may not be realized.
- Treatment must not be for maintenance.
- Reevaluation should occur one time per month or as needed to make changes in the program.
- Occupational therapy services can be reimbursed for designing, fabricating, and fitting orthotic and self-help devices.
- A specific "therapy" diagnosis is no longer required for a beneficiary to be eligible for therapy. Only a demonstrated need for therapy is necessary.
- Therapies are not subject to the intermittence rule and therefore, a one-time-only therapy visit can be made for purposes of safety or instruction.
- Occupational therapy can be provided for patients with psychiatric illness; however, a specific psychiatric diagnosis and the care of a psychiatrist are required. The home care supervisors should be specialized in mental health (Menosky, 1990).

Documentation should always contribute to the overall treatment plan. Keep in mind that under Medicare, therapists are part of a team led by a nurse who may not have much knowledge of our practice. Therefore, our documentation statements must provide her or him with the needed words to establish the plan of care.

Insurance and Home Health Organization Parameters

Some insurance companies and health maintenance organizations (HMOs) follow Medicare guidelines, while others have predetermined the number of visits allowed per year or illness. They may require that documentation notes accompany the billing. In addition, case mangers for the company may also request reports and documentation of the patients. If documentation is not clear, case managers have been known to deny or question an order for activities of daily living training. Muscle reeducation, Cogman exercises, sensorimotor treatment, etc., that bring about functional change in performance areas such as dressing, hygiene, or homemaking are reimbursable.

Contents of Documentation Records

As with all documentation, the records must include identification and background information, assessment and reassessment, treatment planning, and implementation and discontinuation of services. Additionally, in the home, the documentation should pay attention to the components needed for restoration of function. It should address safety and the elimination of permanent loss of abilities. This should be done through the *initial evaluation* that includes tests and evaluations administered and results. It should include a summary and analyses of findings as well as reference to pertinent reports and information. It should also include the occupational therapy problem list and recommendations for services. The treatment plan should include measurable goals, activities, and treatment procedures; type, amount, and frequency of treatment; and the anticipated time required to achieve the goals. There should be a statement of the functional outcomes.

Progress notes must be written for each visit. They must reflect activities, procedures, and modalities used; functional goals; and treatment. They must include the functional assessment of progress as well as response to treatment and progress toward goals related in the problem list. Goal modification should be indicated as well as any changes anticipated in the time required to achieve goals. *Discharge notes* should include a summary of the entire occupational therapy intervention process. Goals achieved and functional outcomes should be stated. A comparison should be made of the initial and discharge status. Home program recommendations and follow-up plans should be made.

Assessment/Evaluation

In the assessment there must be a statement about perceived prognosis; date of onset; prior history and functional status; mental, psychosocial, and emotional condition; as well as environmental, cultural, or architectural barriers. Of course, the assessment of present functional status for activities of daily living, homemaking, or work including sensorimotor, cognitive, and psychosocial deficits or assets is routine. Establishing a baseline testing database at the beginning provides the materials necessary for documenting improvement as change occurs during the course of treatment.

Specific Documentation Guidelines

The following short guidelines will be useful as you prepare your documentation:

- Document the need to employ skilled occupational therapy services.
- Indicate the patient is homebound. Each note must stand alone.
- Put the most pertinent diagnosis first; after that, list all the others.
- Reflect specific clinical observations.
- Do indicate frequency and duration plans at the time of assessment.
- Discharge planning is begun at the time of evaluation.
- Do make your problem list compatible with the master list developed by the care team.
- Document the long- and short-term goals and the discussion of treatment procedures with patient, family, or caregivers.
- Do refer to Uniform Terminology for assistance in structuring the framework for documentation of the strengths and deficits identified in assessment and in identifying those for establishing goals.
- Do establish home programs and make copies for patient's chart.
- Do indicate in notes, instruction to patient, family, and/or caregiver.
- Document all health team conferences, whether they occur by telephone or in person.
- Document changes in treatment plans for reaching the stated goals.
- Change goals to match progress or try new approaches to attain progress.
- Indicate the need for aide, family, or caregiver services in your documentation.
- Slow progress must be justified through documentation that the patient will be able to learn and that the results will eventually result in reduced health care costs.
- Do use cost-effective goal statements.

Be aware that goal statements can often be made into cost-effective goals. For example, a general goal of ability to feed self becomes a cost-effective goal when it is stated: "Patient will become independent in self-feeding so that the home health aide's time may be reduced from 6 hours to 3 hours per day." A goal of training the family in bathing becomes cost-effective when it is stated that the home health aide's time will be reduced by 3 hours. If a patient can become independent in performing toileting, hygiene, and transfers safely; use communication devices; or become capable of using the telephone, a family member may return to work and support the family. This is a cost-effective goal. Goals become cost-effective when the treatment provided is aimed at establishing bed mobility, or ability to reposition self in chair or bed to improve circulation, decrease pain, and prevent decubitus development. Improving patients' functional status and decreasing the amount of work for the spouse may decrease the danger of the caregiver being hospitalized or the potential for both to require nursing home placement. Developing these kind of goals with the nurse or other members of the team can clearly establish the necessity of services.

Documentation Tips

The question is often asked: What should be avoided in the documentation? Or what brings up a "red flag" for a reviewer of Medicare Information Forms? The following examples are problematic but often would not be if more clearly stated.

Avoid the word "maintain." It indicates the patient has reached a plateau; Medicare does not pay for maintenance. A statement such as "treatment was provided to maintain function" should be avoided. If there has been a plateau, and new strategies to reverse the plateau have not been successful in short time, then discharge would be advised. However, a therapist may provide treatment for setting up a maintenance program.

The phrase "making slow progress" should be avoided. The words "steady progress" may more accurately describe the client's progress toward functional goals.

Don't say: "Patient is not progressing." Instead, give the reason why progress has been inhibited. Describe therapist's plan such as "patient placed on hold," or say that changes in goals and treatment were made as a result of the problem.

The word "prevent" must have a connection with the treatment of the condition. For example, the therapist may realize that unless the patient is taught bed mobility there will be decubitus development, or the caregiver may be so taxed that he or she is in danger of hospitalization because of a back or heart problem. It would be better to describe with words that indicate prevention in the following way: The patient is responding to sensory stimulation and neurodevelopmental treatment. He or she has ability to perform 1/4 quarter roll to right. Caretaker reports that now there is decreased redness over coccyx area and indications of increased circulation. Caregiver was provided instruction in back or joint protection techniques decreasing pain and the need for increased aide service. In these instances, evidence of the nurse, therapists, and caregiver working as a team toward goals provides further substantiation of the need for services and shows the patient's increased function and the potential for decreasing cost.

Verbs such as "review, reinforce, or reinstruct" should be used carefully because they make it appear that the service is repetitious or that the patient has been noncompliant or was not able to comprehend.

Avoid the phrase "unable to learn" when there is a learning or cognitive problem. The problem should be addressed indicating goals, treatment techniques, or family or caregiver instructions.

Instead of saying "independent in ambulation using walker" it would be better to say "ambulates with assistance of walker." Care must be taken that documentation statements do not conflict. On occasion a physical therapist will state that the patient is independent with a walker, but the occupational therapist finds that safety is an issue because of loss of balance, perceptual deficit, or impaired safety adherence when attending to other activities such as tasks in the kitchen or bathroom while simultaneously concentrating on ambulation.

Avoid using generalized statements such as "generalized weakness" instead of stating specific functional limitations such as shortness of breath after climbing a few steps; poor balance; or dizzy or unsteady gait. Generalized weakness is usually thought of in conjunction with an illness where intervention is not required to increase strength or where age is the cause of the weakness.

Other generalized statements that are not objective or measurable are "healing well," "responding well," and "good endurance." Be more specific about the changes.

Indicate that the patient is in need of skilled services. Case managers or reviewers may look at training in self-dressing or passive range of motion as nonskilled, seeing it as something that could be administered by untrained personnel or a family member unless there is something in the documentation that shows the uniqueness of your work with the patient. For example, self-ranging may be performed in such a way as to be a part of neurodevelopmental treatment. Dressing may have incorporated proprioceptive neuromuscular facilitation techniques. Backward chaining may be necessary in working with another type of patient, or dressing training may be addressing the perceptual dysfunction.

Duplication of Services

Medicare will not pay for duplication of services. Care must be taken that the documentation proves the disciplines are not duplicating treatments. Transfers training may be done by the physical therapist to determine the level of safety with the technique. The occupational therapist instructs and uses transfer for performance of a daily living skill, such as transfer from wheelchair to bathtub, or wheelchair to toilet with donning and doffing of clothing or toileting hygiene incorporated into this task. The physical therapist may use neurodevelopmental techniques during use of the walker when performing gait training. The occupational therapist may use a similar treatment technique to facilitate increased functional use of the upper extremity in dressing, etc.

In September, 1990 the Health Care Financing Administration (HCFA) issued special instructions regarding dysphagia claims. The new guidelines clarify that occupational, physical, or speech-language therapists can evaluate and treat dysphagia patents and be reimbursed if other coverage guidelines specific to their professions are met (Pinson, 1991). Again, coordination of services with documentation regarding the role of each discipline involved in the case would clarify and prevent problems with reimbursement.

References

Allen, C., Foto, M., Moon-Sperling, T., & Wilson D. (1989). A medical review approach to medicare outpatient documentation. *American Journal of Occupational Therapy 43*, 793-800.

Gillard, M., & Kern, S. (1991, June). *Application of AOTA uniform terminology to practice: Guidelines for documentation.* Paper presented at the American Occupational Therapy Association Conference, Cincinnati, OH.

Menosky, J. (1990). Occupational therapy services for the homebound psychiatric patient. *Journal of Home Health Care Practice, 2*(3), 57-67.

Pinson, C. (1991, February 21). Medicare improvements, Medicaid expansions mark progress. *OT Week*, p. 4.

11. Special Considerations III: Mental Health

Kathleen Kannenberg, MA, OTR/L

This is the last of three chapters discussing special considerations affecting certain areas of practice. The author of this chapter focuses on special documentation problems in the mental health area.

Kathleen Kannenberg is the mental health program manager for the American Occupational Therapy Association.

The health care delivery system has changed dramatically in the past decade. The advent of the Medicare prospective payment system has had a major impact on both publicly and privately funded health programs. Health care consumed approximately 13% of the gross national product in 1991, and that figure is expected to rise (Sawyer, 1991). Increased costs continue to outstrip the national inflation rate (Fine, 1986).

Health care is big business, with large hospital corporations taking over smaller nonprofit and community-based facilities and controlling billions in revenues. The delivery of service that occurs in this highly competitive setting is governed by all the social, economic, and political forces inherent in the business world. The private sector has followed the federal example with development of alternative delivery systems to the traditional fee-for-service base, such as preferred provider organizations, health maintenance organizations, independent practitioners associations, and managed care systems.

Because of the difficulty in defining psychiatric diagnostic categories and quantifying the numerous variables that impact length of stay, Congress provided an exclusionary measure for participation in the diagnosis related group (DRG) system for psychiatric hospitals and general hospitals with psychiatric units. In theory, Medicare, which is the largest payer of occupational therapy services, continues to provide cost-based reimbursement in psychiatry. However, in reality, the reimbursement rate is determined by the Health Care Financing Administration (HCFA), which reviews a hospital's previous year's billing in order to determine a "profile" and then negotiates a per diem amount based on this figure (Novak, 1988).

The managed care systems are designed to provide coverage at a predetermined rate, which is negotiated according to the services desired. Cost containment is the primary influencing factor in the provision of health services. Peer review organizations have been established at both the federal and private levels to provide medical review that monitors use of services in an attempt to cut costs by reducing unnecessary admissions and lengths of stay.

In both systems, if the cost of care is under the predetermined rate, the hospital can keep the difference. But it must also absorb any losses if the cost is higher. This creates a powerful incentive to control costs (Fine, 1986).

The impact of these trends, coupled with the more limited funding available for mental health services, has created a major crisis both for the field of psychiatry and for occupational therapy. The short length of inpatient stays, higher acuity of patients, and rapid turnover have led to significant changes in the focus of mental health care. Treatment approaches emphasize crisis intervention, psychopharmacological intervention, rapid assessment, and early discharge planning.

There is an increasing demand for professional accountability and productivity, stringent cost controls, quality assurance activities, and outcome-oriented treatment (Schwartz, 1988).

The consumers in health care (patients, families, third party payers, health care facilities, industry, and government) are demanding services that provide good value . Because health care dollars must be stretched to cover many providers, questions must be asked about the cost-effectiveness of the treatment provided, e.g., what services the patient received and whether those services were necessary, what the benefit or outcome was for the patient, who is the best provider of these services, and where they should be delivered (Fine, 1986). These outcomes must be measurable and relate to the needs of the consumer.

Ability to Function

But what does the consumer want? The ability to function has been identified as the treatment outcome of greatest interest to the patient (Tarlov, 1983). Research studies have identified adaptive functioning as the second most important factor in determining length of stay for psychiatric patients (Fine, 1988; Mezzich & Coffman, 1985). Hospitals are focusing on containing costs (which lower profit margins) through staffing and budget cuts and increasing opportunities for revenue. Thus there is growing support for improving performance capacities and skills of daily living (Fine, 1988). The American Psychiatric Association has included function (Axis 5) as a component of the medical diagnosis. In its *Diagnostic and Statistical Manual of Mental Disorders* (3rd ed., rev.) (American Psychiatric Association, 1987), the global assessment of functioning scale addresses psychological, social, and occupational function on a continuum of mental health to illness. The scale includes ratings for both current and past year function. The differences in these numbers can provide measurable documentation for rehabilitation potential.

The National Association of Private Psychiatric Hospitals (which includes both profit and nonprofit institutions) has stated that its goal for its patients' treatment is to return patients to optimal functioning and reentry into their activities of daily living to the maximum possible extent. This statement is almost an exact paraphrase of the goal of occupational therapy and, along with the identified needs of other consumers, validates the belief that occupational therapy is in a uniquely advantageous position in the current health care market. Our services are both cost-effective and offer quality outcomes. We must be able to articulate how occupational therapy can meet these consumer needs by speaking a language that has relevance to our audience. Our language is function, and our product is "productive living."

Communication requires that we define and document our role in a way that allows someone who is not an occupational therapist to understand the goals, methods, and outcomes of our services. This is especially a challenge in mental health. Our practice arena is often a centralized "activity or adjunctive therapy" department, which lumps together similar disciplines that use activity as a basis for treatment. From an administrative viewpoint, this centralization provides for cost-effective and coordinated services; the dilemma is that the uniqueness of each discipline can be easily lost. Although disciplines such as occupational, recreation, music, dance, and other creative arts therapies have distinct philosophies, there are many overlap areas, both in scope of services and treatment modalities. This creates role blurring and confusion and often leads to the concept of a generic and interchangeable staff of "activity therapists."

Regulatory bodies, such as the Joint Commission on Accreditation of Healthcare Organizations (JCAHO), Medicare, and state licensing agencies, contribute to this dilemma by defining nonspecific standards for "activity services" that, again, incorporate these disciplines together. For freestanding psychiatric hospitals, there are no specific standards requiring that occupational therapy services be provided.

Another critical factor is the severe shortage of occupational therapists practicing in psychiatry. An American Occupational Therapy Association (AOTA) Member Data Survey in 1973 indicated that 37% of reporting occupational therapists worked in mental health. By 1986, only 22% of therapists identified themselves as mental health practitioners. In 1990, the proportion fell to 17% (AOTA, 1990). Meanwhile, the number of people working in the core professions of psychiatry, psychology, social work, and psychiatric nursing had doubled from 1973 to 1984 (Manderscheid, Witkin, Rosenstein, & Bass, 1984). The number of other professionals working in mental health also increased, with over half of patient care being provided by paraprofessionals (President's Commission on Mental Health, 1987).

The personnel shortage, cost containment, and the prevalence of role blurring have all created an opportunity for other disciplines to fill vacant positions. Unless health care administrators have a clear understanding of the role and value of occupational therapy in meeting consumer demands for functional independence and cost containment, hiring decisions may be based on available personnel, salary requirements, and reimbursement issues.

With all consumers in mental health asking why they should pay for occupational therapy services, what we do that is unique and different from other health care providers, and what is the benefit or outcome of our interventions, it becomes imperative that occupational therapists in mental health communicate their role clearly and with confidence.

Documentation

Documentation in the medical record is the primary format for communicating with both the health care team and third party payers. Reimbursement for services in mental health is an issue regardless of whether your facility includes occupational therapy in the per diem or daily bed rate or bills separately as a fee for service. Whether you practice in an inpatient or outpatient, profit or nonprofit, setting, the highest costs in the mental health delivery system are staffing costs. When administration looks at cost containment, the focus will be on numbers and types of staff as well as the necessity of the services provided in meeting the financial "bottom line." The future of occupational therapy in mental health depends, in part, on our documentation skills.

Psychiatry as a field is struggling with external agency requirements for measurable goals, documented progress, and observable outcomes. Requirements unique to psychiatry that demand a master problem list and goals developed by the multidisciplinary treatment team create broadly based and generic problems and goals.

In trying to meet the requirements for an integrated and multidisciplinary treatment approach, occupational therapists have developed treatment plans that are often ambiguous, difficult to measure, and indistinguishable from other disciplines. Following are three examples of problems (in italics) followed by related goals that might have been written by occupational therapists as well as other members of the multidisciplinary treatment plan.

1. *Depression*: Improve mood, affect, and self-esteem.
2. *Psychotic thought*: Increase reality testing.
3. *Impaired attention span*: Engage in goal-directed activities to increase attention span from 10 to 20 minutes.

In documenting progress, we have documented the process of treatment, the modality provided, what the patient or therapist did, but not the outcome of our intervention and its effect on the patient's functional status. Unfortunately, third party reimbursers and other consumers may not understand how improved self-esteem or attention span contribute to functional outcomes of work, self-care, etc. If we assume this "leap of faith," the uniqueness of occupational therapy's contribution may be lost.

Medicare Guidelines

Why should psychiatric occupational therapists, regardless of their practice setting and reimbursement status, use the Medicare Part B guidelines for outpatient occupational therapy? Because Medicare has the most stringent and specific coverage guidelines, documentation that satisfies Medicare will usually meet the requirements of other third party payers (Acquaviva & Steich, 1988). In addition, Medicare has the only clearly defined criteria for what is considered skilled and nonskilled occupational therapy, and identifies in what circumstances it should be provided and what the outcome of the intervention must be.

By reviewing and understanding the Medicare guidelines for covered services, it becomes clear how we can use the guidelines to document in such a way that our role and value will be clearly delineated and reimbursement will be maximized. The new guidelines were introduced in 1989, following passage of the law that included occupational therapy in Part B, outpatient services. Previously, the only guidelines were for Part A, inpatient services, and these proved to be of limited value for psychiatric occupational therapists, as the following quotation from the *Medicare Part A Intermediary Manual* illustrates:

> Such therapy may involve the planning, implementation and supervision of individualized therapeutic activity programs as part of an overall active treatment program for a patient with a diagnosed psychiatric illness, e.g., the use of sewing activities which require following a pattern to reduce confusion and restore reality orientation in a schizophrenic patient. (HCFA, 1987, p. 3-33.5A)

The new guidelines have a historical significance as it is the first time in the history of HCFA that AOTA has been actively involved in developing standards. The advent of these guidelines has presented our profession with the opportunity to revise our documentation practice in all specialty areas in order to focus on the needs of the patient and the ability to function.

The specific areas in the Part B guidelines that are of primary interest and importance to mental health are highlighted in the following selections (HCFA, 1990).

Cognitive disability is included as a functional limitation in the performance of activities of daily living (ADL). Each level of assistance identified has specific criteria for establishing baseline data and measuring progress:

> §3906.4 A 3. *Moderate Assistance.*—Is the need for 50% assistance by one person to perform physical activities or constant cognitive assistance to sustain/complete simple, repetitive activities safely...The records submitted should state how a cognitively impaired patient requires intermittent one-to-one demonstration or intermittent cueing (physical or verbal) throughout the activity. Moderate assistance is needed when the occupational therapist/caregiver needs to be in the immediate environment to progress the patient through a sequence to complete an activity. This level of assistance is required to halt continuing repetition of a task and to prevent unsafe, erratic or unpredictable actions that interfere with appropriate sequencing. (HCFA, 1990, p. 10-129)

> §3906.2 *Safety Dependence/Secondary Complications.*—A safety problem exists when a patient without skilled occupational therapy intervention cannot handle him/herself in a manner that is physically and/or cognitively safe. This may extend to daily living or to acquired secondary complications...Safety dependence may be demonstrated by high probability of falling, lack of environmental safety awareness, abnormal aggressive/destructive behavior, severe pain....requiring skilled occupational therapy intervention to protect the patient from further medical complication(s). (HCFA, 1990, p. 10-125)

> §3906.4 B. *Change in Response to Treatment Within Each Level of Assistance.*—Significant improvement must be indicated by documenting a change in one or more of the following categories of patient responses within any assistance level:

> 1. Refusals.—The patient may respond by refusing to attempt an activity because of fear or pain. The documentation should indicate the activity refused, the reasons, and how the OT plan addresses them...

> For the cognitively impaired patient, refusal to perform an activity can escalate into aggressive, destructive or verbally abusive behavior

if the therapist or caregiver presses the patient to perform. In these cases, a reduction in these behaviors is considered significant progress, but must be documented, including the skilled OT provided to reduce the abnormal behavior.

For the psychiatrically impaired patient, refusals to participate in an activity frequently are symptoms of the diagnosis. The patient should not be put on a "hold" status due to refusals. If the documentation indicates that the patient is receiving OT, is contacted regularly, and is actively encouraged to participate, medically review the claim to determine if reasonable and necessary skilled care has been rendered.

2. *Inconsistency.*—The patient may respond by inconsistently performing functional tasks from day-to-day or within a treatment session.

Approve the claim when the documentation indicates a significant progression in consistency of performance of functional tasks within the same level of assistance.

3. *Generalization.*—The patient may respond by applying previously learned concepts for performing an activity to another, similar activity. The records submitted should document a significant increase in scope of activities that the patient can perform, their type, and the skilled OT services rendered.

C. *A New Skilled Functional Activity is Initiated.*—Examples:

- Adding teaching of lower body dressing to a current program of upper body dressing;
- Increasing the ability to perform personal hygiene activities for health and social acceptance.

D. *A New Skilled Compensatory Technique is Added.*—(With or without adapted equipment.) Examples:

- Teaching a patient techniques such as one-handed shoe tying;
- Teaching the use of a button hook for buttoning shirt buttons. (HCFA, 1990, pp. 10-130–10-131)

§3906.5 *Level of Complexity of Treatment.*—Base decisions on the level of complexity of the services rendered by the occupational therapist and not what the patient is asked to do. Examples:

A. *Skilled OT.*—The documentation must indicate that the severity of the physical/emotional/perceptual/cognitive disability requires complex and sophisticated knowledge to identify current and potential capabilities. In addition, consider instructions required by the patient and/or the patient's caregivers. Instructions may be required for activities that most healthy people take for granted. The special knowledge of an occupational therapist is required to decrease or eliminate limitations in functional activity performance. Occupational therapists must often address underlying factors which interfere with specific activities. These factors could be cognitive, sensory, or perceptual deficits...

Skilled services include, but are not limited to reasonable and necessary:

- Patient evaluations;
- Determinations of effective goals and services with the patient and patient's caregivers and other medical professionals;
- Analyzing and modifying functional tasks;
- Determinating that the modified task obtains optimum performance through tests and measurements;
- Providing instructions of the task(s) to the patient/family/caregivers; and

- Periodically reevaluating the patient's status with corresponding readjustment of the OT program. (HCFA, 1990, pp. 10-131–10-132)

The Medicare guidelines quoted above have provided psychiatric occupational therapists with a language to identify functional problems and objective criteria to measure and document progress toward independence. As length of stay in acute care has decreased, allowing time only for brief assessment, titration of psychotropic medications, and discharge planning, the occupational therapist's role in providing a safe environment in which to carry out activities of daily living and maximize function becomes more defined.

Writing Goals

Examples of long-term goals (LTG) and short-term goals (STG) that might be written for an acute care setting are as follows:

- LTG 1: Patient will perform basic hygiene and grooming independently by 2 weeks.
- STG 1a: Patient will follow through with one hygiene task (bathe daily) with moderate assistance by 1 week.
- STG 1b: Patient will attend to morning self-care (bathe, comb hair, clean clothes) with minimal assistance by 2 weeks.
- LTG 2: Patient will exhibit personal safety in social conduct with minimal assistance by 3 weeks.
- STG 2a: Patient will verbalize, with minimal assistance, unsafe impulses (set fires, promiscuity) by 1 week.
- STG 2b: Patient will identify safety problems related to impulsive acts, with moderate assistance, by 2 weeks.
- STG 2c: Patient will implement, with moderate assistance, a coping plan to test with therapist impulses that affect her safety in living alone by 3 weeks.

Examples of goals that might be written for other settings include:

- Patient will take a time-out when angry with peers in order to complete a group school assignment, with minimal assistance.
- Patient will initiate social interaction with peers during work break, with moderate assistance.
- Patient's caregiver will demonstrate independence in setting up meal preparation for patient to prepare own lunch.

As occupational therapists in mental health, we should not try to be all things to all people. The view of occupational therapy in psychiatry as providing a generalized therapeutic activity program must be changed. This view diminishes our role as a specialty service for persons with adaptive performance problems and psychosocial rehabilitation needs (Schwartz, 1988). Depending on the patient population and type of facility, we must identify the services that will help our patients to achieve the highest level of function. This may involve our giving up areas that can be done by other professionals, but it will allow us to focus on those skills and interventions that only occupational therapy can provide.

This new format for documentation will require a different way of thinking in order to relate psychiatric problem areas of self-expression, socialization, and mood to functional performance. But isn't that the justification for acute care hospitalization as well as outpatient care—an inability to function effectively at a lower level of care? As we use the levels of assistance to document how progress has been achieved as a direct result of skilled intervention; as we clearly identify the underlying factors and problems that interfere with functional performance; as we establish measurable short- and long-term goals with time frames for accomplishment, our professional boundaries will become clear. The value of occupational therapy in mental health will then be established, both in our own minds and in those of our professional colleagues and consumers.

Dickie (1989) has stated:

> The schism between occupational therapy in mental health and those in other specialty areas narrows or disappears when we talk about reimbursement. Suddenly the language becomes function, and all of us start talking about how to document functional outcomes. Isn't it ironic that third party payers, not necessarily known for their understanding of occupational therapy, are driving this unification of language and purpose? (Dickie, 1989, p. 3)

References

Acquaviva, J., & Steich, T. (1988). Occupational therapy documentation in mental health. In S.C. Robertson (Ed.), *Mental health FOCUS: Skills for assessment and treatment* (pp. 1-169–1-177). Rockville, MD: American Occupational Therapy Association.

American Occupational Therapy Association. (1990). *1990 member data survey*. Rockville, MD: Author.

American Psychiatric Association. (1987). *Diagnostic and statistical manual of mental disorders* (3rd ed., rev.). Washington, DC: Author.

Dickie, V. (1989). From the chair. *AOTA Mental Health Special Interest Section Newsletter, 12*(3), 3-4.

Fine, S. (1986). Trends in mental health. In S. Robertson (Ed.), *Mental health SCOPE: Strategies, concepts, and opportunities for program development and evaluation* (pp. 19-32). Rockville, MD: American Occupational Therapy Association.

Fine, S. (1988). Working the system: A perspective for managing change. *American Journal of Occupational Therapy, 42*, 417-419.

Health Care Financing Administration. (1987). *Medicare part A intermediary manual, part 3: Claims process*. Washington, DC: U.S. Government Printing Office.

Health Care Financing Administration. (1990). *Medicare intermediary manual, part 3: Claims process*. (DHHS Transmittal No. 1487). Washington, DC: U.S. Government Printing Office.

Manderscheid, R., Witkin, M., Rosenstein, M., & Bass, R. (1984). A review of trends in mental health services. *Hospital and Community Psychiatry, 35*, 673-674.

Mezzich, J., & Coffman, G. (1985). Factors influencing length of hospital stay. *Hospital and Community Psychiatry, 36*, 1262-1270.

Novak, E. (1988). Improving payment for occupational therapists in mental health through effective documentation strategies. In *Proceedings: Acute care psychiatry: Practical strategies and collaborative approaches* (pp. 17-25). Rockville, MD: American Occupational Therapy Association.

Sawyer, K. (1991, December 30). Health care spending may reach 14% of GNP. *The Washington Post*, p. A6.

Schwartz, S. (1988). Prospective payment for psychiatric services: Service management strategies for occupational therapy. In S. Robertson (Ed.), *Mental health FOCUS: Skills for assessment and treatment* (pp. 1-37–1-41). Rockville, MD: American Occupational Therapy Association.

Tarlov, A. (1983). The Shattuck lecture: The increasing supply of physicians, the changing structure of the health services system, and the future practice of medicine. *New England Journal of Medicine, 308*, 1235-1244.

President's Commission on Mental Health. (1987). *Final report, volume 1*. Washington, DC: U.S. Government Printing Office.

12. Documentation for Assistive Technology

Aimee J. Luebben, MS, OTR/L

Technology can make a significant difference in the lives of our patients and clients. Patients depend on the occupational therapist not only to suggest appropriate equipment but also to provide the necessary documentation for funding. Documenting the need for equipment, especially expensive high-tech equipment, is a challenge. This chapter provides clear guidance on how to accomplish such documentation, as well as sample letters written to funding sources.

Aimee J. Luebben is the director and assistant professor, occupational therapy program, University of Southern Indiana, Evansville, IN.

Gaining the freedom to be productively employed, participating in recreational activities, caring for personal needs, and living life to the fullest are some of the greatest challenges faced by persons with disabilities. To meet these challenges, technology can serve as an equalizing factor, providing many of the same educational, vocational, self-help, and leisure opportunities available to persons without disabilities (Luebben, 1986).

Although occupational therapy practitioners have been involved with adaptive equipment since the beginning of the profession, assistive technology is relatively new federal terminology. According to The Technology-Related Assistance for Individuals with Disabilities Act of 1988 (PL 100-407), *assistive technology device* means any item, piece of equipment, or product system, whether acquired commercially off the shelf, modified, or customized that is used to increase, maintain, or improve functional capabilities of individuals with disabilities. Most occupational therapy clinicians have recommended specific assistive devices to enhance the quality of life for persons with disabilities, but sometimes the equipment is not funded. The key to funding assistive technology is documentation that is thorough, appropriate, and objective.

In many ways assistive technology documentation is different from the forms of documentation discussed in other chapters. The fundamental difference is the purpose. Documenting services for reimbursement to the person or agency providing occupational therapy services is of prime importance, while documentation for assistive technology is more in the nature of advocacy. Providing funding justification for persons requiring occupational therapy services is the primary purpose for documenting assistive technology needs. Appropriate documentation can assist third party reimbursement sources in making an accurate and informed decision regarding the purchase of adaptive equipment to enhance the lives of persons who need assistive technology.

Another major difference between documenting for occupational therapy services and for assistive technology is the temporal aspect. Most reimbursement requests for occupational therapy services are sent after services have been rendered, while the majority of equipment funding must be preauthorized by the reimbursement source before any equipment can be ordered or delivered.

A third way assistive technology documentation is different from the other forms of documentation is in the variability of documentation. For the most part, when documenting occupational therapy services for reimbursement, a standard format is submitted to the third party payers. However, there is a wide variation in the documentation needed to request financial assistance for assistive technology. The same request submitted to several funding sources may need to undergo several transformations since various funding sources have different requirements for documentation.

Siegel (1991) reported that some clinicians have taken an "ostrich" approach, prescribing equipment based only on clinical parameters and leaving the reimbursement issue to the patient. The frustration inherent in the reimbursement process, the bureaucracy, and arbitrary decisions by the reimbursement sources contribute to further clinician avoidance in becoming involved with the third party payers. If allowed, the justification paperwork for assistive technology can be time consuming and maddening.

Trefler (1989) suggests having a full-time clerical person on staff to direct the funding process; however, with some preparation and insight into the equipment approval process, documentation for assistive technology can be treated as any other type of report writing and generated by the person recommending the device. The precursors to documenting the need for assistive technology are identifying funding sources and using funding strategies. Once a payment source has been targeted and funding strategies employed, the occupational therapy practitioner can write the assistive technology documentation for the person needing the adaptive equipment. For a high incidence of obtaining assistive technology funding, it is essential to follow the funding agency requirements.

Funding Source Identification

One agency may reimburse the total price of an adaptive device, but with expensive equipment, it is becoming more common to combine financial assistance from more than one funding source ("Reimbursing Adaptive Technology," 1989). In order to find funding for specific pieces of assistive technology, it is crucial to know the local availability of funding sources. In every area there is a variety of funding sources including Medicare, Medicaid, private medical insurance, vocational rehabilitation, private and state facilities (e.g., nursing homes, intermediate care facilities for persons with developmental disabilities, sheltered workshops), educational agencies and schools, public fundraising, community service organizations (e.g., Lions, Elks, Variety Club), health organizations (e.g., Muscular Dystrophy Association, United Cerebral Palsy, Easter Seals), and private foundations.

Before approaching a funding source, DeShaw (1990) recommends finding out the rules of the game (whom to contact, what information to present, and how to present the information) and also cautions that the rules for funding sources may change over time, and verification of changes must be made. Knowing specific requirements of the various funding sources can reduce the amount of time spent and paperwork generated. The requirements of federally funded programs and private insurance can vary from state to state, and even missions of service organizations differ locally. Delineating the specifics for each funding group is beyond the scope of this publication; however, two sources that may be purchased are: *The Many Faces of Funding* from Phonic Ear, Inc., 250 Camino Alto, Mill Valley, CA, 94941, 800-227-0735; and *A Road Map to Funding Sources* from the Society for the Advancement of Rehabilitative and Assistive Technology (RESNA), 1101 Connecticut Avenue NW, Suite 700, Washington, DC, 20036, 202-857-1140.

To complete the information regarding available funding opportunities, two other financial options merit exploration: tax benefits and loan programs. Stating that assistive technology is virtually always tax deductible to the individual or business purchaser, Mendelsohn (1991) presents a detailed explanation of specific tax law provisions in the Internal Revenue Code that apply to the purchase of adaptive equipment. If full or partial funding of a device is denied by targeted financial assistance agencies after several appeals, private pay and use of the tax deductibility may prove useful. Planning is the key to use of the tax savings that technology offers (Mendelsohn, 1991).

Various loan programs may provide another option in obtaining assistive technology ("Reimbursing Adaptive Technology," 1989; Rice, 1991). To offer more loan programs, partnerships are being established among combinations of governmental agencies at all levels, funding sources, community agencies, and health organizations. With partnerships sharing some of the costs and risks inherent in providing access to credit, loan programs reduce the expenses of providing financing and arrange to have the lending institution pass savings on to the person who needs financial assistance with assistive technology.

Strategies

While people across the United States are receiving financial support to purchase assistive technology from a variety of funding agencies, other persons with similar disabilities are being denied funding from the same sources for the same adaptive equipment (Pressman, 1987). A theme that is evident from the funding literature is the need for an adviser or advocate, one person who has been designated as the team leader in the pursuit of funding dollars (DeShaw, 1990; Pressman). Other members of the assistive technology assessment and funding-seeking team are all important, but for the most efficient continuity of efforts, one person (a clinician, durable medical equipment dealer, caregiver, or person who is seeking funding for the device) should be named by the team to coordinate each funding search. The advocate becomes the contact person for all involved, compiling information, coordinating communications to funding agencies, and directing necessary cooperative efforts for the team.

In addition to selecting one person to coordinate funding efforts, there are other ways of increasing the likelihood of obtaining funding for assistive technology. Enders (1988) has proposed 10 strategies to assist in receiving financial support to purchase adaptive equipment:

1. Learn the specifics of local service delivery systems that provide funding.
2. Be aware that the entrances to all systems are controlled by gatekeepers.
3. Remember that all funding systems operate within a bureaucratic environment.

4. Request funding in terms consistent with the purpose or mission of the system whose financial assistance is being sought.
5. Be professional in conduct.
6. Educate the funding system on the efficacy of the agency requesting funding.
7. Remember that systems work because of the efforts of the people within them.
8. Remember that all systems have an appeals process.
9. Use external systems to approach the funding systems if needed.
10. Be persistently patient.

Learning the specifics of local service delivery systems that provide funding is the first strategy. Although some funding sources require a large amount of objective documentation, these agencies are not the norm. Many sources prefer a simple justification discussing the equipment and the person. Before wasting needless time and energy on paperwork, the practitioner should talk to a person within the organization to determine the exact needs of the funding agency.

The second strategy is being aware that the entrance to all systems is controlled by gatekeepers. Each agency has specific rules, regulations, and protocols. It is important to take the time to investigate the procedures required to request funding for assistive technology.

To remember that all funding systems operate within a bureaucratic environment is the third strategy. While a bureaucracy can be viewed as an obstacle, this system can work to the advantage of the persons requiring and requesting funding for assistive technology. A bureaucratic hierarchy can be used as a self-contained appeals process if a denial is made at a lower level.

The fourth strategy is to request funding in terms consistent with the purpose or mission of the system from which financial assistance is being sought. The terminology used may make the difference between whether a device receives funding or not.

Hofmann (1990) and DeShaw (1990) have compiled a list of words and phrases used in funding assistive technology with previous success. *Medically necessary, reasonable and necessary, durable medical equipment,* and *prosthetic device* are key phrases for Medicare. Terminology for potential Medicaid and private medical insurance reimbursement includes *achieving and maintaining self-support to prevent, reduce, or eliminate dependency; self-sufficiency; preserving, rehabilitating, or reuniting families; health related; prosthetic appliance; physician-prescribed equipment; part of the client's medical treatment plan;* and *restoration of the patient to his or her best functional level.* For vocational rehabilitation services, successful phrases are *services, training, and equipment used to enhance the employability of the person with a disability; vocational potential; promoting independent living;* and *vocationally enabling.* The reauthorization of PL 94-142, the

Education for the Handicapped Act, as the Individuals with Disabilities Education Act (IDEA) has served to increase special education funding of assistive technology if the multidisciplinary team determines the device to be *educationally relevant, needed in order to receive a free appropriate public education, utilized to facilitate a child's education in the least restrictive environment,* or *providing related services* (Golinker, 1991).

Being professional in conduct is the fifth strategy. Often funding agency personnel never meet the occupational therapy practitioner making the adaptive device recommendation. With many pieces of assistive technology becoming more costly, agencies are cautious about the level of professionalism exhibited by the clinician. Well-written, professional-looking documentation can assist in obtaining funding for adaptive equipment.

The sixth strategy is educating the funding system on the efficacy of the agency requesting funding. Because most funding sources are large bureaucracies, individual staff members often relish the continuity of working with the same clinicians. With a high success rate of determining the most appropriate equipment to meet the needs of the person requiring the device combined with the funding source's conception of purchasing a piece of adaptive equipment that provides value for the money, that funding agency staff person and the clinician are likely to continue having more successes. On the other hand, a clinician without a track record with the reimbursement source may take some time to establish credibility. If literature on the agency requesting funding exists, the clinician should be sure to send it to the funding source.

Meetings prior to requests for funds are also a good way to present the clinician or group of clinicians who will make equipment recommendations. Putting a face to a name often helps the funding agency personnel later when funding is requested. An invitation to provide input to the assessment procedure is always welcomed by the funding agency staff member, though scheduling conflicts often preclude attendance.

To remember that systems work because of the efforts of the people within them is the seventh strategy. To improve the likelihood of receiving funding for adaptive equipment, *Pin Dot News* ("ABCs of Funding," 1990) gives this advice: Write for the reader. Writing for the reader is probably the most important aspect of documenting the need for funding a piece of assistive technology. The person who reads the request may not have an allied health background and may need a more complete explanation of both the device and aspects of the person's disability that warrant recommendation of the piece of adaptive equipment.

The eighth strategy is to remember that all systems have an appeals process. DeShaw (1990) reminds assistive technology funding seekers that denials should not be taken personally, but rather as an indication that a particular funding system is unable to respond to requests at this time. For reimbursement denials, taking a reasoned approach was recommended in a recent article in *OT*

Week ("Claims Denials," 1991), and several tips were given. First of all, for the recommendation that was denied funding, check the documentation. Perhaps there were written aspects that either were unclear or did not receive the emphasis needed for the funding source. After clarifying the language and strengthening the weak points, the practitioner should resubmit the recommendation to the same source. Any communication, including telephone calls, with the funding source should be documented in written form. The record may be used later to show compliance with protocol. If there are repeated denials, the clinician should use the professional network to talk to clinicians who have had similar recommendations funded by the same reimbursement source. Clinicians with funding success may have some insight into the process with that particular agency.

Using external systems to approach the funding systems if needed is the ninth strategy. According to Beck (1991) funds for assistive technology have become increasingly more accessible than in the past, and two ways of solving the funding problem are consumer advocacy and educational efforts. The person for whom the funding is being requested and the family are often key players in the acquisition of funding. If objective documentation justifying the need for equipment fails, often snapshots, videotapes, and letters supporting professional recommendations can change the decision of the funding source in favor of reimbursing for the device.

The tenth strategy is to be persistently patient. This is a key factor. Funding of assistive technology is often a process that is long and filled with obstacles. The practitioner must always remember the person for whom funding is requested. The needs of that person and the improvement in that person's quality of life should supersede the time and effort involved in the process.

Assistive Technology Justification

Proving the need is essential to the acquisition of assistive technology. According to Hofmann (1990) funding requests should contain the following information: a cover letter, the appropriate agency forms, the physician's prescription for the equipment, therapy evaluation(s), and diagnostic reports. When appropriate, pertinent literature describing the device may also be sent.

Often the occupational therapy practitioner has not been designated as the funding advocate, but is responsible only for the justification of equipment. To begin writing the justification, clinicians should remember several points. For the most part, the funding agency staff person reading the documentation and also making the decision regarding the disposition of the equipment may never have met the person with the disability and may be lacking in the background of the disability in functional terms. Appropriate assistive technology justification becomes the link between the current functional picture of the person needing equipment described by the justification writer and the ramifications of the proposed adaptive device and changes in the user's life made by the equipment. In addition, the decision maker is often unfamiliar with the specific pieces of equipment and since there is ongoing change in technology, adaptive device unfamiliarity will continue. Consider the justification an educational process for the reader; describe the device in easily understandable terms and discuss how the equipment will affect the life of the user.

While many therapists once sent lengthy evaluation reports, some clinicians found that a well-written justification in the form of a letter is a welcome substitute for the funding agency. Ideally, the justification should be no longer than two pages and kept to one if at all possible. Even a lengthy justification can be shaped into a two-page document using a new printer that has the ability to select different sizes and shapes of fonts as well as spacing for printing.

To make the best impression on the reader, the justification should be clear, attractive, and free from therapeutic jargon. In a way this piece of documentation is somewhat akin to a sales promotion as the clinician is trying to "sell" the funding source not only on providing financial assistance on the recommended equipment but also on the credibility of the recommendations. A justification written in a professional manner, using correct English, punctuation, and spelling, has a better chance of receiving proper attention by funding agencies.

Since the justification is written in the form of a letter, the salutation is important. For the greatest impact on the prospective funding source, the salutation should greet the reader by name. For the reader, a salutation of "To whom it may concern" may show the need for assistive technology, but it may also be an indication of inadequate follow-through of the team requesting funding assistance. It may take some work to find the exact name of the person in charge of determining funding and to obtain the correct spelling, but the payoff in terms of receiving funding is worth the time and energy expended.

Following the salutation, the justification should contain identifying information (name and birthdate at the minimum) about the person for whom the equipment is being recommended, a statement of the person's diagnosis with a description of the nature of the disability stated in functional terms, a statement regarding the person's abilities, and a prognostic statement regarding the improved ability to function with the device. The prognostic statement can contain information on potential changes in life functioning, e.g., potential maximization, environmental control, independence enhancement, and self-sufficiency improvement.

The next sections should describe the device (model number and company, with address) and discuss the benefits for the person for whom funding is being sought. If there are optional components requested for the device, each piece should have a brief description with a short statement of justification. These individual justification statements for each adaptation, seemingly tedious at the time of writing, may provide necessary information to the decision makers. Unjustified components often result in funding denials that require lengthy appeals.

Several other areas may warrant inclusion in justification documents. Sometimes the funding agency requests that costs be listed in the justification, but often the prices come from another source, the durable medical equipment dealer who was involved in the assistive technology team. Communication with the funding source prior to writing the justification can clarify this issue. Another area that may be included in the justification is a description of the persons comprising the team that evaluated and made the recommendations for the person needing assistive technology. Most funding agencies laud a multidisciplinary evaluation effort with evidence of consumer involvement. Borin (1990) writes that if other pieces of equipment have been tried without success, specific information regarding those devices and the reason for failure should be cited in the justification. This aspect may anticipate questions from funding sources about other equipment available. If equipment had been leased for a trial period, the person's performance with the assistive technology should be documented for the agency making a decision about financial assistance.

A successful formula for the justification is the identification of the person, diagnosis, functional statement, and evaluation team in the first paragraph, with the name of the assistive technology device being requested in the last sentence. The middle paragraphs should contain the individual justification statements for each component of assistive technology being requested. The last paragraph should start by thanking the agency for consideration and assistance, then have a statement describing some possible consequences for the person needing assistive technology if the device is not funded, and end with a name and telephone number to contact if the agency has any questions. The practitioner should complete the justification with a signature and the complete name and credentials (nonabbreviated versions) of the occupational therapy practitioner requesting funding. The clinician should remember to use terminology that is consistent with the funding agency from which financial assistance is being sought.

Following the text in this chapter, several letters are shown that have been successful in obtaining funding for assistive technology. Since funding requirements change from state to state and locale to locale, these documents should be read as guidelines, not copied and used verbatim. Computer technology has assisted in automating justification writing to the point that portions of many of the carefully worded justification documents used in the past may be saved and reused for persons with similar assistive technology recommendations.

An alternative to the justification letter, the Seating/Wheeled Mobility Payment Review Summary, is a form developed by the Specialized Product/Equipment Council through RESNA, an interdisciplinary association for the advancement of rehabilitation and assistive technologies. The form, designed to serve as a communication link between the clinical team and the funding source, summarizes information and organizes evaluation materials and methods (Borin, 1990). Developed to improve the efficiency and effectiveness of the prior authorization system for assistive technology, this form provides a consistent format for concise and complete information regarding the person needing equipment and the adaptive device being recommended by the team. While the Seating/Wheeled Mobility Payment Review Summary deals with only one aspect of adaptive equipment, similar forms using the same format could be developed for other areas of assistive technology. Before using this form or any other formal format, the clinician should check with the funding agency to determine whether the decision makers will accept the form and whether other information will be required.

Conclusion

Two advocacy purposes are accomplished by documentation that is successful in receiving assistive technology financial assistance. First, for the person who needs the adaptive device, the equipment purchased with the requested funds will produce a marked change in his or her quality of life. The second aspect of advocacy is more global in nature. While adaptive devices seem expensive at the onset, assistive technology is proving to be cost saving. Occupational therapy practitioners should not stop communicating with the funding agency after equipment has been approved for funding. Rather clinicians should thank the agency for the needed financial assistance and keep staff members apprised of the user's ongoing progress with the device. This will keep doors open with the funding agency for future requests and also present a current picture of the use of assistive technology. System change occurs more easily at a local level, but clinicians can influence the funding system at the legislative level by showing evidence of successful equipment funding in case studies that have been well-documented to show cost benefits.

References

ABCs of funding. (1990, Spring). *Pin Dot News, 3*(1), 1-2.

Beck, J. (1991). Consumer advocacy: The key to funding. *Communication Outlook, 12*(4), 7-9.

Borin, L. (1990). Documentation for specialized adaptive equipment. *AOTA Developmental Disabilities Special Interest Section Newsletter, 13*(1), 1-2.

Claims denials: Tips on keeping your cool and getting paid. (1991). *OT Week, 5*(7), 9.

DeShaw, D. (1990). Funding issues. *Assistive Technology Information Network, 4*(4), 1-2.

Enders, A. (1988). *The bottom line: Finding funding for technology*. Seminar conducted at the International Conference of the Association for the Advancement of Rehabilitation Technology, Montreal, Canada.

Golinker, L. (1991). *You want us to fund what?* Ithaca, NY: United Cerebral Palsy Associations.

Hofmann, A.C. (1990). The many faces of funding. In B.M. Reid (Ed.), *Branching out in the 90s.* Denver, CO: Colorado Department of Education.

Luebben, A.J. (1986). Low cost high tech: People, equipment, and money resources. In H.J. Murphy (Ed.), *Proceedings of the Second Annual Computer Technology/Special Education/ Rehabilitation Conference, 2,* 225-239.

Mendelsohn, S. (1991). Tax deductibility of assistive technology: A hidden federal subsidy. In H.J. Murphy (Ed.) *Proceedings of the Sixth Annual Conference on Technology and Persons with Disabilities, 6,* 639-648.

Pressman, H. (1987). Funding technology devices. *Exceptional Parent, 17*(7), 48-52.

Reimbursing adaptive technology. (1989, Winter). *NARIC Quarterly, 2*(4), 1, 7-11, 13-15, 17.

Rice, S.R. (1991). Funding assistive technology: Charting the waters of loan programs. In H.J. Murphy (Ed.), *Proceedings of the Sixth Annual Conference on Technology and Persons with Disabilities, 6,* 799-804.

Siegel, J.D. (1991). Strategies for reimbursement. *Proceedings of the Seventh International Seating Symposium: Seating the Disabled, 7,* 263-265.

The Technology-Related Assistance for Individuals with Disabilities Act of 1988, 29 U.S.C. §2201 (1988).

Trefler, E. (1989). The funding challenge for pediatric technology. In *The AOTA practice symposium 1989: Program guide* (pp. 38-42). Rockville, MD: American Occupational Therapy Association.

Figure 12.1 Initial letter requesting adaptive equipment

PL
Crippled Children's Services
Extant, IL

May 8, 1991

Dear PL,

During school annual reviews this year LP, the mother of EP (DOB: 1982), a student with a diagnosis of cerebral palsy resulting in spastic quadriplegia, indicated that the family was having difficulty placing EP in the bathtub and supporting her during her bath. Mrs. Powers asked about the availability of bath chairs. After sending her information with specific measurements, the family decided [on] the Ortho-Kinetics (W220 N507 Springdale Road, P.O. Box 436, Waukesha, WI 53187, 800-558-7786) 52-inch TLC bath chair (#6741) with waterproof headrest (#6701-01). In addition to utilizing the device for its intended purpose, the family will also use the bath chair for an extra positioning device both in the house and in the yard during nice weather.

Mrs. P also inquired about the adaptive toilet chair utilized in the classroom. As part of her classroom programming, EP uses a stand alone child sized potty chair for toilet training and has been most successful. To ensure continuity and also decrease the need to buy expensive diapers, I recommend that she have the same system at home. The chair is a wooden and metal chair manufactured by Rifton, Route 313, Rifton, NY, 12471, 914-658-3141. Recommended are E82, Large Child's Potty Chair; E822, Backpad; E817, Footrest with seven inch sandals; and E861, tray. All components may be found on page four of the 1990/91 Rifton catalog.

Thank you for your assistance in this matter. The bath chair and potty chair will afford safety and optimal positioning during bathroom tasks. If you have any questions, please contact me at the above number.

Sincerely yours,

Aimee J. Luebben, MS
Licensed Occupational Therapist
Certified Educator

Figure 12.2 Initial letter requesting augmentative communication device

KB
Community Club
King Road
St. Louis, MO

February 13, 1991

Dear KB,

In the course of speaking with you in the last few years, I have mentioned that I will be coming to you sometime in the future to ask for funding on a speech prosthesis for a very deserving person. CA (DOB: 1973) is the young man I have been speaking about and he is now ready to have his own RealVoice augmentative communication device.

CA has a diagnosis of cerebral palsy resulting in spastic quadriparesis. So motorically involved that he is unable to speak and has little reliable, voluntary movement, CA makes laughing noises at jokes so we know that intelligence is locked inside his body. One day, when we first got the computer at school and provided access for CA, we found that he knew his colors, shapes, letters, and numbers, all of which had been untestable in the past. For the last two years CA has been using my RealVoice two days a week when I am scheduled to be in his facility and a flashlight when the RealVoice is unavailable. In the classroom he now makes requests by utilizing the RealVoice.

There is excellent followup at home. CA's mother is a teaching assistant in an early childhood classroom and his sister, TA, is working while going to school to become an early childhood teacher. They report CA is much more relaxed at home than at school and is able to accomplish some complex motor movements. With the consistent success we have had at school, we had a team meeting of teacher, teaching assistants, speech pathologist, and therapists and decided CA was ready for his own device. After consultation with the speech pathologist, we recommend that CA have a similar system for his own use. Available from Adaptive Communication Systems (800-247-3433) and recommended are a RealVoice (male) with the light board placed in a pan that fits over the keyboard, a light pointer, and a Quick and Easy Mount to attach the system to his wheelchair. His wheelchair is new and was funded through CHAMPUS, but this insurance does not fund communication devices.

His mother, LA, is aware there is an application process for Community Club funding process and eagerly awaits your information. Thank you for your assistance in this matter. With a speech prosthesis, CA will not only gain a "voice," but also will be more independent and have some control over one aspect of his life. If you have any questions, please contact me at the above number.

Sincerely yours,

Aimee J. Luebben, MS
Licensed Occupational Therapist
Certified Educator

JR
Crippled Children's Services
Extant, IL

April 10, 1990

Dear JR,

JF of Rehab Medical; JO, Physical Therapist; BT, Physical Therapist Assistant; and I evaluated CH (DOB: 1974) for a seating and mobility system. CH has a diagnosis of cerebral palsy resulting in right spastic hemiparesis and, because of her physical limitations, requires assistance for all activities.

Her current system consists of an Everest and Jennings standard manual wheelchair with Otto Bock lateral supports, heel loops, lap belt, and lap tray. Since the Pin Dot prefabricated contour seat did not provide adequate positioning, it was removed and she is now sitting on a piece of egg crate foam, but assumes a windswept posture with her hips twisted and trunk flexed laterally to the other side. At the last clinic her physician prescribed that CH wear her body jacket all day. Although she wears it at school, compliance with the wearing of the orthosis at home is inconsistent. Because CH has the functional use of one arm, independent propulsion for mobility of a standard wheelchair is difficult and slow.

Recently CH had a trial use of a Meyra one hand drive (left) mobility system. As soon as she was placed in the chair, she was able to propel herself independently and was learning to fine tune maneuvers such as turning and backing up. This same Meyra system we recommend for mobility.

The seating system is more easily assessed by separating the back from the seat component. We recommend a Jay Back with deep lateral supports that will accommodate CH during the times when she is wearing the orthosis and when she is not. A Danmar chest harness will assist in providing circumferential type pressure at the trunk when the orthosis is removed. She has been positioned in just about every other type of planar, hybrid, and prefabricated contour seat available; positioning was unsatisfactory in each case. For this reason we recommend a contour seat, custom fabricated for CH.

Since her feet move around in the standard foot plate with figure eight straps, a more aggressive system, shoe positioners/channels, is recommended for CH. We recommend a laptray for anterior upper extremity support and a surface for fine motor activities, and a hip strap mounted at 45 degrees of the hip angle to position her correctly in the chair.

Thank you for your assistance in this matter. With a one arm drive mobility system CH will gain more independence and control of her life; the seating system will provide support for postural integrity and decrease the potential for surgical procedures. If you have any questions, please contact me at the above number.

Sincerely yours,

Aimee J. Luebben, MS
Licensed Occupational Therapist
Certified Educator

LS
Medical Social Consultant
Crippled Children's Services
High Street
Nemo, IL

August 29, 1990

Dear LS,

JF of Rehab Medical and I evaluated JC (DOB: 1971) on July 23, 1990 with JC's mother, a caregiver, and two people from UCP present during the assessment. JC is currently not using a wheelchair. He has been unable to tolerate his current planar type manual push wheelchair and was placed on homebound status in his school district since he screamed when placed into his old wheelchair. JC has a diagnosis of cerebral palsy resulting in spastic quadriplegia. He currently has no method of positioning and desperately needs a new wheelchair.

JC's muscle tone is increased and a strong asymmetrical tonic neck reflex interferes with positioning. Secondary to hypertonia JC's range of motion is limited; he has fixed deformities of the hips, shoulders, knees, and elbows and tightness in other joints. Little voluntary movement was observed; however, it was noted that when the seating system was completed, JC relaxed his fisted hands.

Because of his severe deformities and physical limitations, a standard, planar seating system is not reasonable or appropriate and a contour seating system custom molded to his body is needed for proper support. He was fitted in a molding frame adjusted to accommodate the few degrees of trunk flexion he has. The Comfi back and seat cushions are Contour U components which will be fabricated from soft supportive material from the molds made of JC on site.

While the molds of the seating system were custom molded during the assessment, the mobility unit was researched and carefully selected since the seating system approximates a full reclining position. A Motion Designs Zippie Tilt wheelchair was chosen, and the 14 inch wide seating system will fit between the bars of the 16 inch frame. The tilt mechanism is recommended because, with the presence of primitive reflexes, it is necessary to angle JC in space to provide position changes and shifts in weight bearing areas. The standard Zippie seating system was deleted and trunion and pan components will be used to attach the seating system to the mobility unit.

Thank you for assistance in this matter. A new wheelchair will provide necessary support to assist in maintaining JC's remaining postural integrity. If you have any questions, please contact me at the above number.

Sincerely yours,

Aimee J. Luebben, MS
Licensed Occupational Therapist
Certified Educator

Figure 12.5 Initial letter requesting van modifications

PL
Crippled Children's Services
Extant, IL

December 12, 1990

Dear PL,

CC (DOB: 1987) has recently been fitted with a standard type wheelchair in a child's size. As you recall, CC has a diagnosis of cerebral palsy resulting in spastic diplegia and is dependent on others for her self care needs. The family has purchased a minivan, but needs financial assistance in obtaining a lift for the van. To promote safety in moving CC into and out of the family's transportation system as well as during travel, I recommend the van be modified by professionals to include a lift and the appropriate wheelchair tiedowns.

Thank you for your assistance in this matter. If you have any questions, please contact me at the above number.

Sincerely yours,

Aimee J. Luebben, MS
Licensed Occupational Therapist
Certified Educator

BJ
Nursing Consultant
Crippled Children's Services
High Street
Nemo, IL

January 16, 1990

Dear BJ,

LY, Physical Therapist, JF of Rehab Medical, and I evaluated HE (DOB: 1975) for a new seating and power mobility system. As you know he has a diagnosis of high level spinal cord injury and is outgrowing his present system which has not proven reliable in terms of mobility.

Because HE is unable to manually operate a wheelchair, we recommend another powerdrive wheelchair, a narrow adult model with an 18 inch seat depth. He must recline at various times during the day to shift his weight and prevent costly skin breakdown; for this a tilt and zeroshear recline mechanism is recommended for HE.

To access the mobility and recline mechanisms, recommended are the following: a joystick mount, a short throw chin joystick with appropriate hardware and electronics, and a dual function recline interface. The interface mounting kit will be mounted on a bib and will not swing out of HE's range as his current system does. HE needs a ventilator and battery tray with adaptor mounts to support his various supportive apparatus and two batteries for his use.

For the seating system HE is positioned well in an extra long Jay cushion with adductor pads, hip guides, and an abductor. The Jay is a hybrid cushion which provides the proper support while assuring skin integrity via flotation gel. An Otto Bock headrest with multiaxis offset hardware and headrest adaptor mount will provide support for his head and two large scoliosis pads with left and right support hardware will align his body within the narrow adult wheelchair.

A buckle seat belt mounted at 45 degrees to the angle of his hips will keep HE back in the wheelchair, and an acrylic tray will provide necessary anterior upper extremity support. To position his feet properly, angling footplates and velcro straps are needed.

Thank you for your assistance in this matter. If you have any questions, please contact me at the above number.

Sincerely yours,

Aimee J. Luebben, MS
Licensed Occupational Therapist
Certified Educator

JR
Crippled Children's Services
Extant, IL

July 24, 1991

Dear JR,

I understand Illinois Medicaid has placed a ceiling dollar amount on specific seating adaptations. In a letter dated April 22, 1991 I outlined specific recommendations for a seating system for MS (DOB: 1986) who has outgrown his Orthokinetic travelchair. According to the dealer, Rehab Medical, Medicaid has allowed limited funding for three specific pieces of equipment: a biangular back, trunk laterals, and Danmar harness. This letter is written to clarify why these specific wheelchair adaptations were recommended and to reiterate the medical necessity of these particular devices.

MS has a diagnosis of cerebral palsy resulting in spastic diplegia and he prefers sitting in his current wheelchair with his back in a rounded position. This is causing a reversal of the normal curves of his back and is also promoting scoliosis. If this process is not retarded, MS will require costly surgical procedures for correction. The biangular back is designed to assist MS in sitting up straight and to discourage leaning over. The laterals recommended for his trunk are more expensive as they are curved. The curved devices are stronger and decrease the potential for skin breakdown. Since we have already tried the harness that meets the Medicaid dollar amount without success as the straps move off his shoulders during bus transportation, the Danmar chest harness, a one piece design that can be bent to fit MS's chest shape, was recommended.

Thank you for your assistance in this matter. In all of our recommendations we try to provide the optimal positioning for the best value, and as Illinois tax payers, we are mindful of the costs involved. The three specific pieces of equipment are the ones that are needed to provide support for postural integrity, decrease the potential for surgical procedures, and allow safety during transportation. If you have any questions, please contact me at the above number.

Sincerely yours,

Aimee J. Luebben, MS
Licensed Occupational Therapist
Certified Educator

13. Using the Concurrent Review Form

Cathy Crispen, MA, OTR/L

It is usually difficult to review our own notes and look for omissions. Very often we know the content too well to see what is missing. This author presents a form developed by occupational therapy medical reviewers in California to correspond to Medicare Part B guidelines, the most stringent reimbursement guidelines. It is, therefore, an excellent tool to review your own notes or those of others. Use it on several charts of discharged patients. Have you documented the important information? What have you written that is not necessary? See if you consistently miss the same information. It can be a valuable tool for enhancing your documentation.

Cathy Crispen was formerly payment manager for the American Occupational Therapy Association and is currently the regional director of occupational therapy, Nova Care, Northeast Division.

After a patient has received occupational therapy services and the appropriate documentation has been completed, the service provider then sends the payer the bill for those services. The payer may then elect to complete a medical review to ensure that the occupational therapy services billed were actually covered by the policy or coverage guidelines. In many instances, to complete the medical review, the payer requests the documentation from the provider of the services. This documentation is then reviewed for two purposes: technical accuracy and medical necessity. Claims are paid or denied based upon both the accuracy and appropriateness of the therapist's documentation.

When reimbursement is denied or delayed, it is frequently due to insufficient documentation or clerical errors. It is recommended that the therapist should take time to review the claims and documentation before they are sent to the payer to screen the material for errors or incomplete documentation material.

The Concurrent Review Form

The guidelines and Concurrent Review Form (CRF) presented in this chapter are to assist therapists in providing the proper documentation and patient information necessary for a fair review of their claims to any payment source. Figure 13.1 on the opposite page shows a typical patient information sheet, while Figure 13.2 (placed at the end of the text in this chapter) shows the CRF used by Blue Cross of California. *All references in this chapter to numbered items on the CRF are references to Figure 13.2.*

Payers such as Medicare, Medicaid, worker's compensation, and private insurance companies have personnel that perform the review of therapy claims. A majority of the reviewers are not occupational therapists; they are nurses or other professionals. Payers have varied criteria or guidelines for reviewing their claims; currently, the most stringent are the Medicare Part B medical review guidelines.

In an effort to expedite the review process and ensure consistent judgment among several reviewers, Blue Cross of California, Medicare Medical Review Division, has developed a CRF for its staff to use when reviewing occupational therapy claims. This form contains the elements upon which a determination can be made on the payment of a claim. It can be used to review any therapy documentation for any payer. The CRF will be used throughout this chapter to assist therapists in reviewing their own as well as their peers' documentation. If the therapist's documentation has the elements present to meet or exceed the criteria on the CRF, then it is most likely that the documentation meets or exceeds the standards of a majority of payers.

Technical Aspects

The first step in a medical review and in a peer review is to check the claim for the correct patient information (technical requirements). A review of the "technical" requirements (a Level 1 Review for Medicare purposes) typically includes verifying the *International Classification of Diseases—9th Revision* (ICD-9) diagnosis code(s) that correlate with the diagnosis that is related to the occupational therapy service rendered. The ICD-9 diagnosis codes

Figure 13.1 Patient information sheet

MEDICARE OUTPATIENT PART B
Therapy Billing Information
(OT, SP, IT, PR, CR)

Item 10 - Patient's Name: **Smith, Margaret**
Last, First

Item 22 - Billing Period: **08/13/88 - 09/13/88**

Item 28 - Occurence Code: **11** Onset Date: **06/21/87**
Onset diag. reported in item 77

to

Item 33 - Occurence Code: **35** Start of Care Date: **7/13/88**
Date initial therapy began

Item 51 - Revenue Code: **430** (OT-430, SP-440, IT-412, PR-948, CR-943)

Item 52 - Visits **11**
Actual number of visits this billing period

Item 68 - HIC: **123   45   6789A**
Patient's Health Insurance Claim number

Item 77 - Primary Diagnosis: **Multiple Sclerosis**
Diag. must substantiate why therapy is being given

ICD-9 CODE: **340**

Therapist: **OTR** Date: **10/18/88**

are frequently found on the patient's medical chart, can be obtained from the physician, or are listed in the ICD-9-CM code manual (U.S. Department of Health and Human Services, 1989). The first or primary code that is listed on your therapy claim should be for the primary patient problem for which you are providing therapy. You may list a secondary code if there is an additional problem that relates to occupational therapy. If a diagnosis code is listed that pertains to the medical treatment of the patient, such as ICD-9 code 599.0 (urinary tract infection), and not the problem necessitating therapy, such as ICD-9 code 342.1 (spastic hemiplegia), the claim could be denied because the patient does not require skilled occupational therapy.

The technical review also includes verifying the onset date for the occupational therapy treatment diagnosis and the date of the start of the occupational therapy care. Only in rare instances should these dates be the same. The onset date should precede the start of care date (see Figure 13.1).

The number of treatment visits should also be listed on the bill. If the initial evaluation visit(s) fall within that billing period, those should appear in the visit total. Frequently, the number of procedures given during the visit is mistaken for the number of actual visits. This causes the number of visits to appear excessive for that billing period (see Figure 13.1).

This information corresponds to the patient information sheet and items 1 and 2 on the CRF. Often billing or medical records clerks complete the above technical information on patient claims. They may misunderstand the therapist's documentation or have a lack of experience in coding. It is important that the therapist check the claims for accuracy; these errors cause a substantial delay in processing the claim because the payer must request additional information before performing a final review. If the technical requirements are met on the claim, the payer goes on to review the actual documentation to determine the "medical necessity" of the claim. This documentation may be provided in an attachment to the bill or the medical record.

Medical Necessity Aspects

A review of the documentation for occupational therapy services typically includes the following:

- a physician's referral when required
- a physician's certification when required
- an initial evaluation that includes a summary of the patient's medical history
- daily notations of the therapy visits
- monthly and/or weekly progress notes
- an itemized statement of the daily therapy charges
- an Occupational Therapy Functional Assessment Report (OTFA)

If you use the CRF to analyze your documentation for appropriate content and completeness of information, you may avoid the submission of deficient documentation.

Physician's Order

The therapy records should include a written physician's order if it is required by the payment source. The complete order should include the occupational therapy treatment diagnosis, the onset date of the diagnosis, the request for evaluation and/or specific treatment orders, an estimation of frequency and duration, the date, and the physician's signature. If the physician makes a referral for services, the therapist should establish a treatment plan outlining the type of activity or procedure(s) and the frequency and duration of that treatment, with the therapist's signature and the date, at the time of the initial evaluation. Any changes or additions to this plan by the therapist or physician must be in writing, should be signed and dated, and should appear in the record. If the physician writes specific treatment orders, they must be followed unless the therapist receives a written change in orders by the physician (see CRF 3a).

Frequency and Duration

Frequency and duration of therapy are estimates by the therapist about the patient's potential to successfully attain the therapy goals within the prescribed time. The *frequency* (times per week) and *duration* (length of treatment program) must be specific rather than a span of time, e.g., three times per week for 4 weeks (see CRF 3b). If the initial estimate of either the frequency or duration proves to be inappropriate during the course of therapy, an adjustment can be made by documenting the change in either the progress notes or the monthly plan of care (physician certification).

Physician Certification

Payers such as Medicare, Part B, and Medicaid require *certification* for therapy services. This is a statement written by the therapist and agreed to by the physician, indicating that the patient needs occupational therapy services. This certification is valid for 30 days from the initial evaluation date or for 30 days from the previous certification. Many payers accept the initial written physician's order as the first certification. Most payers require that the signature be in writing, not a stamp or computer generated (see CRF 3c, 5, and 6).

Certification or recertification may be placed on a form provided by the payer or one developed by the therapist, but it should contain the following elements:

- a statement that is written or checked off indicating that the physician has seen the patient during the 30-day certification period (if required by the payer)
- a statement of need for continuing therapy
- specific frequency and duration of treatment
- a statement that the physician will review the plan every 30 days (if required by the payer)
- the physician's signature and date
- the therapist's signature and date

Initial Evaluation

Documentation should include an *initial evaluation*. Within this record should be information to substantiate the need for skilled occupational therapy intervention. The patient's medical history should be detailed, with an emphasis on the patient's prior level of function (see CRF 4). The record should also contain baseline physical and cognitive data, in both subjective and objective form, that relate to the functional recovery of the patient. The data can be obtained in various ways and should be specific to the patient's diagnosis and functional problems.

The trend of many payers is to follow Medicare's lead in wanting verification that the patient and/or caregiver was interviewed concerning the activities performance the patient seeks to accomplish from the therapy, e.g., independence in dressing or minimal assistance in homemaking tasks (see CRF 7a). Payers also want evidence that the therapist observed the patient perform specific functional activities and determined the baseline functional level (see CRF 7b and e, and 10d). If the therapist notes a possible need for adaptive equipment, environmental adaptation, or instruction in compensatory techniques, there should be a correlation with the identification of factors that are interfering with the performance of the task, such as decreased range of motion, perceptual deficits, inability to access areas of the home due to confinement to a wheelchair, etc. (see CRF 7c and d).

Long-term goals should be listed. They should be goals that the patient is expected to have accomplished at the end of the occupational therapy treatment program (see CRF 7f). Short-term goals that are related to the accomplishment of each long-term goal should also be outlined. The short-term goals need to be broken down into activities that can be accomplished within that monthly billing period (see CRF 7g).

Goal statements should contain two parts: the *functional outcome statement* and the *enabling intent*. A functional outcome statement identifies the desired patient performance resulting from therapy. Enabling intent identifies the method by which a therapist enables a patient to accomplish the stated goal.

Notations and Progress Notes

Many payers, such as Medicare, require that each patient visit be documented with a notation. At a minimum, this documentation should include the date of treatment, the length of the session, the activity or procedure, and any changes that occur in the patient's progress.

These daily notations are then used to write the required weekly and/or monthly progress note (see CRF 8). The progress note should document changes in the patient's performance of the stated goals from the beginning of the notation period to the end. Relevant underlying factors such as pain, a change in medication, or a change in behavior or ability to follow instruction should be related to the activity performance and noted in the documentation. If a patient accomplishes a goal, it should be noted and that goal deleted from the list. If a goal is not reached, an explanation should be provided. It may be necessary to modify the unaccomplished goals due to inappropriateness, lack of patient interest in working on that particular activity, or the exacerbation of underlying factors (see CRF 8, 9, and 11).

Upon discharge from therapy, a discharge summary becomes a final progress note. It should summarize progress on goals throughout the course of treatment and also include any training given to caregivers, home program instruction, and equipment issued to the patient. Further need for occupational therapy services should be described as well as any follow-up that will occur.

Occupational Therapy Functional Assessment Report

Often therapists are required to supply an OTFA report on their patients to attorneys, worker's compensation boards, employers, schools, physicians, and other health care settings. These reports provide a means of making decisions regarding the patient by persons who are not occupational therapists or even health care professionals. Reports should be written with the specific audience in mind and the reason(s) for which the report was requested. The audience for whom the OTFA report is written is often not familiar with occupational therapy jargon and abbreviations, and these should be avoided. Common definitions of words should be used as well as simplified descriptions, instead of terminology that is unique to the profession, as in *Uniform Terminology for Occupational Therapy* (2nd ed.) (American Occupational Therapy Association, 1989). The documentation format most commonly used in the OTFA report is narrative. The report contents are organized into three or four sections: introduction/history, findings, interpretation, and recommendations/summary. The report should be typewritten, single-spaced.

Other Requirements

To partially fulfill the requirements of some federal and state regulations that there be a demonstration of adequate supervision of certified occupational therapy assistants (COTAs), it is recommended that notes written by COTAs be cosigned by an occupational therapist. This is a requirement of Medicare's Conditions of Participation as well as of many state occupational therapy licensure regulations. It is wise to confirm the requirements for your particular setting.

Frequent Reasons for Denial of Claims

The most frequent cause of denial is that the service the therapist performed is not covered by the policy, plan, or guidelines. There could be several reasons why the services given by the therapist are deemed noncovered by the payer, including the following numbered examples:

1. The documentation does not demonstrate that a *skilled* occupational therapy service was provided. The treatment must have a certain level of complexity that can only be performed safely and effectively by an occupational therapist or COTA under the supervision of a therapist. If the patient or a caregiver could provide the documented care (e.g., daily feeding program, repetitive range of motion exercises, endurance activities, daily practice in activities of daily living) or another service could provide the same care, then skilled occupational therapy may be unnecessary (see CRF 10a, b, c).

2. The documentation does not show that there was *significant practical improvement and progress* on the patient's goals in a reasonable amount of time. If the patient has not sustained gains, the therapy is considered to be at a maintenance level or not reasonable for the expectations set. Therapists need to document movement in levels of assistance and/or improved patient response to assistance given (see CRF 8, 9, 10 and 11).

3. The documentation fails to establish that the patient with a specific diagnosis would not improve naturally without the intervention by occupational therapy. At times, the typical progression of the medical condition would spontaneously return the patient to normal function. Occupational therapy may be necessary when there are extenuating circumstances that would hinder that spontaneous recovery. That information

must appear in the documentation for consideration; otherwise the payer will assume that the treatment was not "necessary" for that particular diagnosis.

4. Some payers, due to restrictions in their policies or guidelines, only pay for certain types of occupational therapy services in certain therapy settings. Your documentation may be excellent, but the patient might not be covered for your services. It is recommended that insurance policies and payer guidelines be reviewed on a regular basis for restrictions or changes in coverage. Medicare coverage remains stable for long periods, but Medicaid, private insurance, and worker's compensation coverage change frequently. Private insurance policies vary from individual to individual and are the most difficult to track.

5. A majority of payers will only pay for *direct service provision*. They usually do not pay separately for the therapist to attend case conferences, staffings, or inservices. They also will not accept billing for separate documentation time by the therapist. The expectation is that these activities will be part of the cost of the treatment time and built in to that charge (see CRF 10e).

Conclusion

It is the therapist's responsibility to demonstrate that the occupational therapy service provision is reasonable and necessary for that particular patient. The payers cannot make interpretations or suppositions based on information not present in the record. Again, it is recommended that the therapist screen the claims for accuracy and take the time to review documentation before it is sent to the payer. Provision of inservices to the appropriate billing clerks and medical records personnel may be useful in decreasing billing errors for occupational therapy claims. By following the CRF guidelines, therapists should be able to provide documentation to the payers that includes all of the elements necessary to establish medical necessity for that occupational therapy service.

Exercises

In order for you to gain an understanding of the use of the CRF in reviewing your documentation, case studies of actual occupational therapy claims are reviewed on the pages following Figure 13.2. It must be understood that there is no right or wrong way to review documentation. Also, for specific diagnoses, not all elements of the CRF may need to be present in the documentation. Two reviewers looking at the same documentation may see very different elements present. This form is only a tool to assist the therapist and reviewer to look systematically at documentation.

Case A is a claim for occupational therapy services for a female inpatient in a psychiatric facility. Case B is a claim for occupational therapy services for a female patient in a skilled nursing facility. Both claims are complete from initial evaluation to discharge from therapy. When reviewing the documentation for Cases A and B, note the different documentation styles and formats as well as the ease or difficulty in locating the elements listed on the CRF. After reading the cases reviewed by the author, turn to Case C and use the CRF to review the documentation yourself. Note that the patient in Case C had not yet been discharged when this record was pulled; therefore, no discharge summary is present.

At the very end of this chapter, after the case material, there are some follow-up questions that highlight several important issues.

References

American Occupational Therapy Association. (1989). *Uniform terminology for occupational therapy* (2nd ed.). Rockville, MD: Author.

U.S. Department of Health and Human Services. (1989). *International classification of diseases, 9th revision, clinical modification* (3rd ed.). (DHHS Publication No. PHS 89-1260). Washington, DC: U.S. Government Printing Office.

Figure 13.2 Concurrent Review Form

Concurrent Review of Outpatient Occupational Therapy Services

1. Primary diagnosis: _____ Onset date: _____

2. Treatment diagnosis: _____ Onset date: _____

Documentation includes the following:	YES	NO	COMMENTS
3. Treatment plan	Yes	No	
a. Written physician order specifically states the modality or procedure to be performed.	Yes	No	
b. Specific frequency and duration of treatment.	Yes	No	
c. Certification is timely. From: ____ To: ____ Date: _____	Yes	No	
4. Prior functional level.	Yes	No	
5. How long has the patient been treated since the initial OT evaluation? Date of evaluation: _____ Length in days: 30 60 90 120			
6. Is therapy going to continue after this billing period? Why?	Yes	No	
7. Initial patient evaluation record includes: a. Initial interview with patient and/or caregiver about activity performance and services requested/needed.	Yes	No	
b. Observation of patient's activity performance (functional performance).	Yes	No	

	YES	NO	COMMENTS
c. Identification of adaptive equipment, environmental adaptation, or compensatory techniques needed.	Yes	No	
d. Identification of underlying factors interfering with task performance that are therapeutic indications for occupational therapy (e.g., ROM, strength, perceptual and/or cognitive problems, etc.).	Yes	No	
Awareness of hazards:			
Impaired sensation	Yes	No	
Impaired comprehension	Yes	No	
Impaired perception	Yes	No	
Impaired attention span	Yes	No	
Impaired strength	Yes	No	
Incoordination	Yes	No	
Abnormal muscle tone	Yes	No	
Limitations in ROM	Yes	No	
Impaired body scheme	Yes	No	
Perceptual deficits	Yes	No	
Impaired balance/head control	Yes	No	
Environmental barriers	Yes	No	
Inadequate psychosocial resources	Yes	No	
e. Objective functional limitations identified in therapist's documentation? (Problem list)			
Functional activities	Yes	No	
Assistance levels			
Physical	Yes	No	
Cognitive	Yes	No	
Response to within assistance levels	Yes	No	
Assistive device/equipment	Yes	No	
f. Long-term goals identified?	Yes	No	
g. Short-term goals identified?	Yes	No	
8. Are there weekly *objective* measures of patient progress or problems in achieving treatment goals?	Yes	No	

Requested/Needed Activities	Date Assistance/Response	Date Assistance/Response	Date Assistance/Response
Eating			
Feeding			
Grooming—hygiene			
Bathing			
Dressing			
Writing skills			
Homemaking skills			
Avocational skills			
Transfers (toilet, tub)			
Mobility—wheelchair			
Activity tolerance			
Equipment–assistance/ adaptive devices			
Joint protection			
Energy conservation— work simplification			
Object manipulation			
Assistance requesting skills: Attendant, family, public			
Money management			

	YES	NO	COMMENTS
9. Does documentation address stated problems as per treatment plan?	Yes	No	
10. Is Medicare being billed for noncovered services?	Yes	No	
a. *No skilled OT.*	Yes	No	
i. Routine exercises	Yes	No	
ii. Routine assistance with self-care activities	Yes	No	
iii. Endurance training	Yes	No	
b. *Maintenance care* (slow or no progress).	Yes	No	
i. Sawtooth loss–gain: Unable to sustain gain, no overall improvement	Yes	No	

c. *Duplication* of services with PT, ST, Neuropsychologist, or RN.	Yes	No	
d. Evaluation as a *screening* device.	Yes	No	
e. *Deleted* services?	Yes	No	
i. Case conferences	Yes	No	
ii. Billing separate documentation time	Yes	No	
iii. Billing for reevaluations that were not ordered	Yes	No	

11. Was the patient discontinued from occupational therapy when one of the following criteria was met?

_____ a. Achieved goals.

_____ b. Has reached a plateau in progress (slow or no progress).

_____ c. Unable to participate in the treatment program because of medical, psychological, or social complications.

_____ d. Treatment no longer requires skilled OT (i.e., can be continued by patient or caregivers).

This form is courtesy of Blue Cross of California. Adapted with permission.

Concurrent Review of Outpatient Occupational Therapy Services

1. Primary diagnosis: major depression with   Onset date: no indication
   psychotic features, bipolar-mixed

2. Treatment diagnosis: paranoia   Onset date: no indication

Documentation includes the following:	YES	NO	COMMENTS
3. Treatment plan	Yes	No	
a. Written physician order specifically states the modality or procedure to be performed.	Yes	(No)	Form not signed by M.D.
b. Specific frequency and duration of treatment.	(Yes)	No	Gave a range—not specific
c. Certification is timely. 12/8/88 12/24/88 From: ✓ To: ✓ Date: _____	(Yes)	No	
4. Prior functional level.	Yes	No	Unable to secure or maintain employment (chronic)
5. How long has the patient been treated since the initial OT evaluation? Date of evaluation: 12-8-88 Length in days: (30) 60 90 120			
6. Is therapy going to continue after this billing period? Why?	Yes	(No)	Discharge note present
7. Initial patient evaluation record includes:			
a. Initial interview with patient and/or caregiver about activity performance and services requested/needed.	(Yes)	No	
b. Observation of patient's activity performance (functional performance).	(Yes)	No	

	YES	NO	COMMENTS
c. Identification of adaptive equipment, environmental adaptation, or compensatory techniques needed.	Yes	(No)	
d. Identification of underlying factors interfering with task performance that are therapeutic indications for occupational therapy (e.g., ROM, strength, perceptual and/or cognitive problems, etc.).	(Yes)	No	
Awareness of hazards: Impaired sensation	Yes	No	
Impaired comprehension	Yes	No	
Impaired perception	Yes	No	
Impaired attention span	(Yes)	No	*preoccupied*
Impaired strength	Yes	No	
Incoordination	Yes	No	
Abnormal muscle tone	Yes	No	
Limitations in ROM	Yes	No	
Impaired body scheme	Yes	No	
Perceptual deficits	(Yes)	No	*poor judgment*
Impaired balance/head control	Yes	No	
Environmental barriers	Yes	No	
Inadequate psychosocial resources	(Yes)	No	
e. Objective functional limitations identified in therapist's documentation? (Problem list)			
Functional activities	Yes	(No)	*These do not appear in problem/goal list.*
Assistance levels Physical	Yes	(No)	
Cognitive	Yes	(No)	*Impairments appear on enclosed evaluation form. Not addressed until discharge note.*
Response to within assistance levels	Yes	(No)	
Assistive device/equipment	Yes	(No)	
f. Long-term goals identified?	(Yes)	No	
g. Short-term goals identified?	Yes	(No)	
8. Are there weekly *objective* measures of patient progress or problems in achieving treatment goals?	(Yes)	No	

Requested/Needed Activities	Date 12/14 Assistance/Response	Date 12/22 Assistance/Response	Date 12/24 Assistance/Response
Eating	not listed	not listed	I
Feeding			I
Grooming—hygiene			I
Bathing			I
Dressing			I
Writing skills			
Homemaking skills			
Avocational skills			
Transfers (toilet, tub)			I
Mobility—wheelchair			I
Activity tolerance			
Equipment–assistance/ adaptive devices			
Joint protection			
Energy conservation— work simplification			
Object manipulation			
Assistance requesting skills: Attendant, family, public			requires assist
Money management			

	YES	NO	COMMENTS
9. Does documentation address stated problems as per treatment plan?	(Yes)	No	
10. Is Medicare being billed for noncovered services?	Yes	No	not clear from records
a. *No skilled OT*.	Yes	No	
i. Routine exercises	Yes	No	
ii. Routine assistance with self-care activities	Yes	No	
iii. Endurance training	Yes	No	
b. *Maintenance care* (slow or no progress).	Yes	No	
i. Sawtooth loss–gain: Unable to sustain gain, no overall improvement	Yes	No	

c. *Duplication* of services with PT, ST, Neuropsychologist, or RN.	Yes	No	
d. Evaluation as a *screening* device.	Yes	No	
e. *Deleted* services?	Yes	(No)	
i. Case conferences	Yes	No	
ii. Billing separate documentation time	Yes	No	
iii. Billing for reevaluations that were not ordered	Yes	No	

11. Was the patient discontinued from occupational therapy when one of the following criteria was met?

_____ a. Achieved goals.

_____ b. Has reached a plateau in progress (slow or no progress).

_____ c. Unable to participate in the treatment program because of medical, psychological, or social complications.

_____ d. Treatment no longer requires skilled OT (i.e., can be continued by patient or caregivers).

_____ ✓ _____ Was discharged from facility

This form is courtesy of Blue Cross of California. Adapted with permission.

Document A

GENERAL OBSERVATIONS	Intact	Impaired	Comments
Grooming		✓	bizarre dress - sunhat
Affect		✓	flat
Reality Orientation		✓	x2, confused
Memory		✓	unreliable historian
Activity Level		✓	hyperactive
Thought Process/Content of Speech		✓	paranoid
Self-Concept		✓	low

INTERPERSONAL BEHAVIOR	Intact	Impaired	Comments
Independence		✓	
Cooperation	✓		
Socialization		✓	seclusive, lacks skills
Expression of Anger		✓	
Expression of Feelings		✓	internalizes

TASK PERFORMANCE	Intact	Impaired	Comments
Attn. Span/Concentration (30 min.)		✓	10 min. pre-occupied
Fine Motor Coordination	✓		
Decision-Making	✓		
Ability to Follow Directions		✓	1 step, requires refocusing
Attention to Detail		✓	
Organizational Skills		✓	requires external structure
Impulse Control	✓		
Frustration Tolerance	✓		
Problem-Solving		✓	requires assistance
Interest in Activity		✓	engages, lacks interest

FUNCTIONAL SKILLS			
Activities of Daily Living (age appropriate)	Intact	Impaired	Comments
Self-Care		✓	has skills, does not
Money Management		✓	initiate
Transportation		✓	
Meal Planning & Preparation		✓	
Home Management		✓	
Safety & Health		✓	poor judgement

Ingleside Hospital
Rosemead, California

**REHABILITATION SERVICES
OCCUPATIONAL THERAPY
EVALUATION SUMMARY AND TREATMENT PLAN**

PAtient # 00300

FUNCTIONAL SKILLS (cont).
Time Management:

	Intact	Impaired	Comments
Ability to Structure Productively		✓	lacks self gratification
Balance of Work and Leisure		✓	imbalance
Identifies Interests/Aptitude		✓	isolative
Awareness of Community Resources	✓		
Ability to Utilize/Follow Through		✓	

Occupational Role: __unemployed__
  Ability to Function __unable to secure or maintain employment (chronic)__

Precautions/Contraindications __none indicated__
Diagnosis (Axis 1) __Major Depression w/ Psychotic features R/O Bipolar, mixed__
Patient Goals __refused to identify__
Referral Recommendations __none__
Comments __Patient was cooperative w/interview, but guarded in disclosing personal information.__

OCCUPATIONAL THERAPY RECOMMENDATIONS/TREATMENT PLAN

It is felt that ___patient name___ is appropriate for and would benefit from the Occupational Therapy treatment program. The patient will be seen in occupational therapy for __1-2__ hour(s), __5-6__ time per week, or as tolerated, in small groups/individual treatment sessions. Treatment will continue for the duration of hospitalization, unless otherwise indicated by a physician order.

PROBLEM	GOAL
① Paranoia	① increase frequency & length of interactions with others
② Psychotic thought & behavior	② improve ability to sustain attention to task & conversation
③ Dysphoric Mood	③ increase spontaneous expression of affect

METHOD

- ___ one to one
- ✓ living skills
- ✓ task skills
- ___ prevocational/vocational

- ✓ communication/self expression
- ___ health education
- ✓ sensory motor
- Other: _____

Date of Evaluation __December 8, 1988__ Therapist _____ __MA, OTR__

Treatment Program Approved _____
                                                        Physician

[H] Ingleside Hospital
Rosemead, California

REHABILITATION SERVICES
OCCUPATIONAL THERAPY
EVALUATION SUMMARY AND TREATMENT PLAN

Patient # 00300

ATTENDANCE CODE

Document B

✓ = Attended   R = Refused
E = Excused   O = Did not attend

Attendance from ___December 8___ to ___December 14 1988___

OCCUPATIONAL THERAPY TREATMENT	MON	TUES	WED	THURS	FRI	SAT	SUN
Evaluation				compl KRK ✓	✓	✓	
Task skills							
Living skills							
Communication/self expression				O	✓		
Prevocational/vocational							
Health education							
Sensory motor							
One to one							✓ R
Other							

DATE __Dec. 14/89__ OT Weekly Progress Note

Patient is consistent in group attendance, responding to a kind firm approach, despite her paranoia. She is a passive group participant, observing from the periphery of the group. Problems!

1) Paranoia — Patient displays a decrease in paranoia, as demonstrated by improved eye contact and ability to respond briefly to approach. She is reluctant to engage in process, but has made the first step of attendance.

2) Psychotic thought + behavior — She continues to demonstrate psychotic thought process, as seen by her apparent responses to internal stimuli and continued difficulty sustaining attention. She does respond to refocusing and is able to work for brief periods on simple tasks.

3) Depressive Mood — She continues to appear depressed, as seen by her flat affect and seclusiveness. It is difficult to determine progress on depressed mood —→

Patient # 00300

DATE

12/14/88   because of her paranoia.

Plan

Continue to implement current OT treatment
plan, with special emphasis on developing a
rapport & providing structure that supports reality.

JTR

PATient # 00300

ATTENDANCE CODE

Document C

✓ = Attended   R = Refused
E = Excused   O = Did not attend

Attendance from **Dec 15** to **Dec 22, 1988**

OCCUPATIONAL THERAPY TREATMENT	MON	TUES	WED	THURS	FRI	SAT	SUN
Evaluation							
Task skills	✓		✓	✓	✓		
Living skills					✓		
Communication/self expression		✓		✓			
Prevocational/vocational							
Health education							
Sensory motor		✓				✓	
One to one							
Other							✓

DATE 12/22/88   OT Weekly Progress Summary —
Patient is attending groups regularly and requires only minimal reminders to participate.

1) Paranoia — Although she continues guarded and is minimally self-disclosive, she displays increased trust and is able to respond to longer interactions with both peers and staff. Posture continues rigid.

2) Psychotic thought & behavior — Her behavior is increasingly reality oriented ie although she continues to wear summer clothes in winter, she will take off her sunhat while in group. She is occasionally distractible and pre-occupied, but is no longer responding to hallucinations. She is oriented x3 now.

3) Dysphoric mood — Her mood continues depressed. Affect remains flat and when in unit milieau, she remains withdrawn from peers. She does not verbalize any feelings, needs, although she will respond to task oriented questions. ————→

Patient #00300

DATE
12/22 | Cont.

Plan continue current OT plan. Focus on depressed mood, by initiating one to ones to support verbalization of feelings.

—OTR

ingleside hospital

Rosemead, California

UNIFIED PROGRESS NOTES

#00300

Case A *(continued)*

Document D

ATTENDANCE CODE

✓ = Attended   R = Refused
E = Excused   O = Did not attend

Attendance from __12/22__ to __12/24/88__

OCCUPATIONAL THERAPY TREATMENT	MON	TUES	WED	THURS	FRI	SAT	SUN
Evaluation							
Task skills	✓						
Living skills							
Communication/self expression		✓					
Prevocational/vocational							
Health education							
Sensory motor		O					
One to one							
Other		D/C					

DATE 12/24/88 OT Discharge Summary

Patient participated regularly in groups during her hospitalization. Participation within group process continued passive & required facilitation.

Initial OT goals —

1) increase frequency & length of interactions
2) improve ability to sustain attention to task & conversation
3) increase spontaneous expression of affect

Goals 1 & 2 were met; goal 3 unmet due to patients' chronic paranoia and limited length of stay. She demonstrated increased trust + ability to engage w/others. Only minimal reminders were required to elicit group attendance and she was able to dress appropriately at time of discharge.

Her speech, although minimal in content and length, was goal directed and she was able to request needs in an appropriate manner. She continued to appear depressed. Affect brightened minimally in

#00300

Effective Documentation for Occupational Therapy

DATE
12/24 response to group involvement. She was not able to spontaneously interact, but was responsive to approach. Interest level in activities improved only slightly, although she was able to verbalize positive feelings related to accomplishments. Self esteem, continued low.

Master Treatment Plan Problems:
Problems 1, 2, and 5 were addressed in the OT treatment plan + progress is indicated above.
Functional Abilities + Deficits:
Patient requires external structure and support to organize + follow-through on basic activities of daily living. Within this structure, she is able to carry out self care, but requires assistance in all other areas. She would benefit from a structured living environment which would provide the support required for her to maintain in the community.

K. _____ OTR

UNIFIED PROGRESS NOTES

Concurrent Review of Outpatient Occupational Therapy Services

1. Primary diagnosis: IT Fx neck of femur—left   Onset date: 12-20-88

2. Treatment diagnosis: Same   Onset date: Same

Documentation includes the following:	YES	NO	COMMENTS
3. Treatment plan	Yes	No	
a. Written physician order specifically states the modality or procedure to be performed.	(Yes)	No	not signed by MD
b. Specific frequency and duration of treatment.	(Yes)	No	5x/week for 1 mo.
c. Certification is timely. From: 1-3-89 To: 3-3-89 Date: _____	(Yes)	No	
4. Prior functional level.	(Yes)	No	Independent
5. How long has the patient been treated since the initial OT evaluation? Date of evaluation: 1-3-89 Length in days: 30 (60) 90 120			
6. Is therapy going to continue after this billing period? Why?	Yes	(No)	discharge note present
7. Initial patient evaluation record includes:			
a. Initial interview with patient and/or caregiver about activity performance and services requested/needed.	(Yes)	No	
b. Observation of patient's activity performance (functional performance).	(Yes)	No	

	YES	NO	COMMENTS
c. Identification of adaptive equipment, environmental adaptation, or compensatory techniques needed.	(Yes)	No	
d. Identification of underlying factors interfering with task performance that are therapeutic indications for occupational therapy (e.g., ROM, strength, perceptual and/or cognitive problems, etc.).	(Yes)	No	
Awareness of hazards: Impaired sensation	(Yes)	No	hearing
Impaired comprehension	(Yes)	No	ST memory
Impaired perception	(Yes)	No	judgment, problem solving
Impaired attention span	Yes	No	
Impaired strength	(Yes)	No	
Incoordination	Yes	(No)	
Abnormal muscle tone	Yes	(No)	
Limitations in ROM	(Yes)	No	
Impaired body scheme	Yes	(No)	
Perceptual deficits	Yes	No	mild
Impaired balance/head control	Yes	(No)	
Environmental barriers	Yes	(No)	
Inadequate psychosocial resources	Yes	(No)	
e. Objective functional limitations identified in therapist's documentation? (Problem list)			
Functional activities	(Yes)	No	
Assistance levels Physical	(Yes)	No	
Cognitive	Yes	(No)	
Response to within assistance levels	Yes	(No)	
Assistive device/equipment	(Yes)	No	
f. Long-term goals identified?	(Yes)	No	
g. Short-term goals identified?	(Yes)	No	
8. Are there weekly *objective* measures of patient progress or problems in achieving treatment goals?	(Yes)	No	

Requested/Needed Activities	Date 1-6 Assistance/Response	Date 1-13 Assistance/Response	Date 1-20 Assistance/Response
Eating			
Feeding			
Grooming—hygiene	√ mod/max	√ min	√ occ. min to I
Bathing	√ min		
Dressing	√ UE mod/min LE max	√ UE min LE max/mod	√ LE mod UE min ↑ within level
Writing skills			
Homemaking skills			
Avocational skills			
Transfers (toilet, tub)	√ mod/max X 2	√ mod/max X 1	√ SBA X 1
Mobility—wheelchair		√ mod	√ min
Activity tolerance			
Equipment–assistance/ adaptive devices	√	√ adapt. equip for dress.	√
Joint protection			
Energy conservation— work simplification			
Object manipulation	√	√	√
Assistance requesting skills: Attendant, family, public			
Money management			

	YES	NO	COMMENTS
9. Does documentation address stated problems as per treatment plan?	(Yes)	No	
10. Is Medicare being billed for noncovered services?	Yes	No	not apparent
a. *No skilled OT.*	Yes	No	
i. Routine exercises	Yes	No	
ii. Routine assistance with self-care activities	Yes	No	
iii. Endurance training	Yes	No	
b. *Maintenance care* (slow or no progress).	Yes	No	
i. Sawtooth loss–gain: Unable to sustain gain, no overall improvement	Yes	No	

c. *Duplication* of services with PT, ST, Neuropsychologist, or RN.	Yes	No	
d. Evaluation as a *screening* device.	Yes	No	
e. *Deleted* services?	Yes	No	
i. Case conferences	Yes	No	
ii. Billing separate documentation time	Yes	No	
iii. Billing for reevaluations that were not ordered	Yes	No	

11. Was the patient discontinued from occupational therapy when one of the following criteria was met?

_____ ✓ _____   a. Achieved goals. — pt. discharged to home

_____   b. Has reached a plateau in progress (slow or no progress).

_____   c. Unable to participate in the treatment program because of medical, psychological, or social complications.

_____   d. Treatment no longer requires skilled OT (i.e., can be continued by patient or caregivers).

This form is courtesy of Blue Cross of California. Adapted with permission.

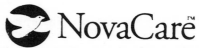

NovaCare™ OCCUPATIONAL THERAPY EVALUATION DATA

Patient's Name	Birth Date	Sex F	Eval Date: 1/3/89

Facility Boulder Manor Room _____ Medicare # _____ Co-Insurance # _____

Diagnosis IT Fx Neck of Femur (L) Onset Date 12/20/88 Physician _____

Previous OT None

Medical Hx Osteoarthritis (B) shoulders
obesity

UPPER EXTREMITY (R) Hand dominant

RT	LT	AREA	ACTION		RT ROM	LT		RT INTACT	IMPAIRED	LT INTACT	IMPAIRED
3	2⁺	shoulder	flex	extend	120/30	90/10	Coordination	X		X	
2⁺	2	shoulder	abd	add	110/90	100/90	Muscle Tone	X		X	
2⁺	2⁺	shoulder	int rot	ext rot	50/60	50/55					
3	3⁻	elbow	flex	extend	WNL	WNL					
3	3	forearm	sup	pro			Contracture	None			
3	3	wrist	flex	extend			Tremor	None			
3⁺	3	hand			↓	↓	Pain	4/0 (L) Hip pain ; (B) shoulder			

16# 14# grip   pain upon movement

COGNITION	INTACT	IMPAIRED	SENSORIMOTOR	INTACT	IMPAIRED
Orientation	X		Vision	X c̄ glasses	
ST Memory		X mildly	Visual Tracking	X	
LT Memory	X		Hearing		X HOH
1 Step Command	X		Body Scheme	X	
2 Step Command	X		Motor Planning	X	
Judgement		X safety	R/L Discrimination	X	
Attention Span	X		Spatial Relations	X	
Problem Solving		X	Sequencing	X	
Receptive Language	X				
Expressive Language	X			RT	LT

ORAL MOTOR	INTACT	IMPAIRED	SENSATION	RT int	imp	LT int	imp
Tongue Movements	X		Lt Touch	X		X	
Chewing	X		Temperature	X		X	
Swallowing	X		Proprioception	X		X	
			Stereognosis	X		X	

ACTIVITIES OF DAILY LIVING (IND – independent; SUP – supervised; VQ – verbal cueing; MIN – minimum physical assist; MOD – moderate physical assist; MAX – maximum physical assist; U – unable; NT – not tested).

Feeding IND	Grooming MOD	Oral Care MIN	Toileting MAX x 2
U/E Dress MOD	L/E Dress U	Fasteners IND	Bathing NT
Bed Mobility MAX x 2	Sitting Balance 4⁻/5	Transfers MAX x 2	Ambulation NT
W/C Mobility U	Endurance 2/5		

Equipment W/C Ted hose

Precautions NWB (L) L/E ; SOB upon exertion

Prior level of function Lived alone in Sr. Apt. complex ; (I) in self-care, functional

Add Comments mobility. 3 meals/day provided along c̄ housekeeping
                    & laundry services

          – supportive family ; pt & family motivated for d/c home

REHAB POTENTIAL Good for stated goals

GOALS 1) ↑ grooming/oral care to (I) 2) ↑ U/E dressing to min, L/E dressing to mod (A)
3) ↑ func. xfers to max x 1 4) ↑ w/c mobility to mod (A) 5) ↑ (B) U/E strength, ROM
to 3⁺/5   LTG: (I) self-care ; d/c home

RX PLAN self-care trng., functional mobility trng., assess for & train in use of
adaptive equipment, (B) U/E therapeutic exercise

FREQ OF RX 5x/wk · 6 wks AMT 45-50 DUR up to THERAPIST'S SIG _____ OTR
          then 3x/wk   2 months

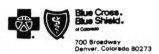

Blue Cross.
Blue Shield.
of Colorado

700 Broadway
Denver, Colorado 80273

FORM APPROVED
OMB NO. 0938-0233

Medicare Rx For Prescription Therapy Only
Initial – Part A

PHYSICIAN USE THIS FORM TO PRESCRIBE: ☐ PHYSICAL THERAPY (P.T.) ☒ OCCUPATIONAL THERAPY (O.T.)
☐ SPEECH PATHOLOGY (S.P.)

COMPLETE THE FOLLOWING TO ASSURE PROPER MEDICARE REIMBURSEMENT

BENEFICIARY NAME | AGE: 84

BENEFICIARY ADDRESS (Street, City, State, Zip Code) | HEALTH INSURANCE CLAIM NO.

PRIMARY DIAGNOSIS (conditions for which therapy is prescribed)
IT Fx Neck of (L) Femur 820.21

DATE OF ONSET OF PRESENT CONDITION
Month 12 | Day 20 | Year 88

SECONDARY DIAGNOSIS (bearing on condition therapy)
osteoarthritis (B) shoulders 715.01

DATE PATIENT FIRST RECEIVED THERAPY FOR CURRENT CONDITION
Mo. 01 | Day 03 | Yr. 89

WAS SURGERY PERFORMED FOR PRIMARY DIAGNOSIS? ☒ YES ☐ NO (If "Yes," indicate nature of surgery and date)
ORIF

Mo. 12 | Day 21 | Yr. 88

ASSESSMENT OF REHABILITATION POTENTIAL
Good for stated goals

GOALS OF TREATMENT PLAN
1) ↑ grooming/oral care to (I) 2)↑ u/e dressing to min, 4/e to mod (A) 3)↑ functional xfers to max (A) x 1 4)↑ w/c mobil. to mod (A) 5)↑ (B) u/e strength, ROM to 3⁺/5 LTG:(I) self-care s/c home

PRESCRIPTION (agents and techniques ordered — indicate changes or variations)
Eval
self-care trng., functional mobil. trng., assess for & train in use of adapt. equip.
(B) u/e therapeutic exercise

ORDERED FREQUENCY OF TREATMENT
5x/wk

NUMBER OF TREATMENTS ORDERED
20-25

DURATION OF TREATMENT PROGRAM
1 month, renewable

HAS PATIENT RECEIVED PRIOR ☐ P.T. ☒ O.T. ☐ S.P. FOR SAME CONDITION? ☐ YES ☒ NO (If "Yes," give location and date)
LOCATION | DATE

PROGRESS SUMMARY INCLUDING PERTINENT MEDICAL INFORMATION AND SIGNIFICANT CHANGES
Pt. was living alone in apt. in Sr. Complex, (I) in basic ADL's, when she fell & fractured hip. Eval. results indicate pt. requires mod (A) grooming & u/e dressing (unable to participate in 4/e dressing 2° pain), max (A) x 2 functional mobility. (B) u/e function ranges from 2-3⁺/5. Pt. is currently NWB (L) 4/e. Judgement/problem solving skills are mildly impaired. Skilled O.T. indicated to ↑ pt's. functional (I) for d/c home.

*See attached eval

COMPLETED BY | TITLE: OTR | DATE 1/3/89

PHYSICIAN NAME | PHYSICIAN SIGNATURE (required only when used as prescription)

PHYSICIAN ADDRESS (Street, City, State, Zip Code) | DATE

WHITE/Provider File — CANARY/Billing (attach to HCFA 1500 or UB-82/HCFA 1450) — PINK/Physician — GOLDENROD/Provider Working File

FORM NO. 99318 (REV. 1-85)

Attn. Nursing: 1/3/89

To transfer

1) requires max Ⓐ of 2 people
2) she is non-weight bearing on
   her left leg
3) transfer her to her right side;
   remove right armrest & legrest
   from w/c prior to transfer

Any ?'s - contact

- O.T. or
- PT

THANKS !

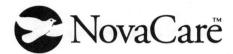NovaCare™

FOURTEEN DAY PROGRESS REPORT

PT   (OT)   ST

Patient:_____Physician_____

Initial Tx. Date: <u>1/3/89</u>   Facility: <u>Boulder Manor</u>

Today's Date: <u>1/17/89</u>   Tx. to Date <u>Eval + 10</u>

Diagnosis: IT Fx Neck of (L) Femur
          Osteoarthritis (B) shoulders

Goals: 1)↑ grooming/oral care to (I)
        2)↑ U/E dressing to min, L/E to mod (A)
        3)↑ func. xfers to max (A) x1
        4)↑ w/c mobility to mod (A)
        5)↑ (B) U/E strength. ROM to 3⁺/5

Progress:
    Grooming/oral care has ↑ from min/mod (A) to (I). U/E
dressing has imp. from mod to min (A); L/E from unable
to mod/max (A) + use of adapt. equip. Func. xfers have
imp. from max (A) x2 to mod max (A) x2. w/c mobility
skills have imp. from unable to min/mod (A) up to
50'. (B) U/E grip strength ↑ from 16# to 19#, (L) from 14# to
16.# Pt. voicing fewer c/o (B) shoulder pain during ADL
tasks.

Plan: Cont tx 5x/wk. Goals: 1)↑ dressing to min (A) 2)↑ func.
xfers to min/mod (A) 3)↑ w/c mobility to (I) 4)↑ (B) U/E strength/.
ROM to 3⁺/5

☒   Please sign and return

_____   _____ OTR
        Physician   Therapist

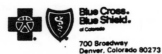

Blue Cross.
Blue Shield.
of Colorado

700 Broadway
Denver, Colorado 80273

Re-cert 2/2-3/4/89

FORM APPROVED
OMB NO. 0938-0233

Medicare Rx For Prescription Therapy Only

PHYSICIAN USE THIS FORM TO PRESCRIBE: ☐ PHYSICAL THERAPY (P.T.) ☒ OCCUPATIONAL THERAPY (O.T.)
☐ SPEECH PATHOLOGY (S.P.)

COMPLETE THE FOLLOWING TO ASSURE PROPER MEDICARE REIMBURSEMENT

BENEFICIARY NAME | AGE
84

BENEFICIARY ADDRESS (Street, City, State, Zip Code) | HEALTH INSURANCE CLAIM NO.

PRIMARY DIAGNOSIS (conditions for which therapy is prescribed)
IT Fx Neck of (L) Femur   820.21

DATE OF ONSET OF PRESENT CONDITION
Month 12 | Day 20 | Year 88

SECONDARY DIAGNOSIS (bearing on condition therapy)
Osteoarthritis (B) shoulders   715.01

DATE PATIENT FIRST RECEIVED THERAPY FOR CURRENT CONDITION
Mo. 01 | Day 03 | Yr. 89

WAS SURGERY PERFORMED FOR PRIMARY DIAGNOSIS? ☒ YES ☐ NO (If "Yes," indicate nature of surgery and date)
ORIF
Mo. 12 | Day 21 | Yr. 88

ASSESSMENT OF REHABILITATION POTENTIAL
Good for stated goals

GOALS OF TREATMENT PLAN
1) ↑ dressing to (I) c̄ adapt. equip. 2) ↑ functional mobility to (I) 3) ↑ u/e strength ROM to 3⁺/5 4) ↑ toileting to (I) 5) D/c home

PRESCRIPTION (agents and techniques ordered — indicate changes or variations)
self-care trng (dressing, toileting, bathing), functional mobility trng; trng. in use of adapt. equip., therapeutic exercise, home assessment / d/c planning

ORDERED FREQUENCY OF TREATMENT
5x/wk 2 wks, then 3x/wk 2 wks

NUMBER OF TREATMENTS ORDERED
18

DURATION OF TREATMENT PROGRAM
1 month

HAS PATIENT RECEIVED PRIOR ☐ P.T. ☒ O.T. ☐ S.P. FOR SAME CONDITION? ☐ YES ☒ NO (If "Yes," give location and date)

LOCATION | DATE

PROGRESS SUMMARY INCLUDING PERTINENT MEDICAL INFORMATION AND SIGNIFICANT CHANGES
Pt. has made significant gains in tx. u/e dressing imp. from mod (A) to (I), u/e from unable to min/mod (A), toileting from max (A) x 2 to mod (A) x 1, w/c mobility from unable to (I) 150'. Pt. is now PWB (L) u/e (as of 2/1/89). (B) u/e shoulder ROM has imp. an average of 10° each movement; grip strength has ↑'d from 16# to 20# on the (R); from 14# to 17# on the (L). Skilled O.T. necessary to further ↑ functional (I) for d/c home.

COMPLETED BY | TITLE OTR | DATE 2/2/89

PHYSICIAN NAME | PHYSICIAN SIGNATURE (required only when used as prescription)

PHYSICIAN ADDRESS (Street, City, State, Zip Code) | DATE

2/24/89

Dressing Sequence

* Before beginning, gather necessary items (clothing, adaptive equipment). Sit in chair with walker in front of you.

Undressing
1. Remove shirt, bra
2. Stand up. Pull slacks & panties down to knees. Sit down.
3. Using reacher, unhook Velcro tabs on shoes. Remove shoes using dressing stick.
4. Use dressing stick to remove slacks, panties.
5. Use dressing stick to remove socks.

Dressing
1. Put on bra, shirt
2. Use sock aid to put on socks.
3. Use dressing stick to put on panties, slacks (put left foot in 1st). Pull up over knees.
4. Use shoehorn to put on shoes
5. Stand up. Pull up panties, slacks.

_____, OTR

Patient Name: _____

~~Do circled exercises~~ _10_ times each, _2_ times daily.

Do each exercise slowly and completely, breathing normally
DO NOT HOLD YOUR BREATH!

Sitting or Lying Down:

① Shoulder flexion: Start with hands in front of you, lift arms up over head.

② Abduction: Arms straight out to the sides, bring arms out and together overhead.

③ Arms straight out to sides, bring hands together in front of you.

④ Touch hands to shoulder, then up toward ceiling.

⑤ Bend and then completely straighten elbows.

⑥ Try to bring hands together at back of neck, then at the low back.

⑦ Elbow bent, arm at side, turn palm up and down.

⑧ Circle wrists.

⑨ Open and close hands.

⑩ Bring fingers apart or together.

⑪ Circle thumbs.

_____ OTR

3/1/89

Home Program — Bathing

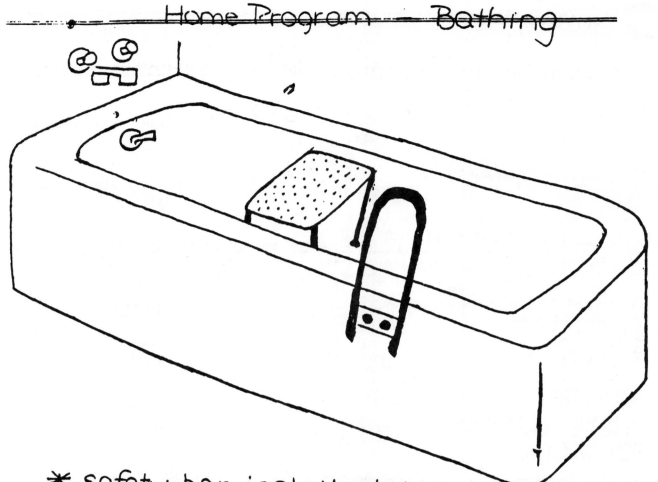

* safety bar installed behind tub bench
* use longhandled sponge when bathing

Entering Tub :
   1) turn walker and back up toward tub
   2) using safety grab bar, sit down
   3) turn and lift feet into tub

Exiting Tub :
   1) While sitting, turn (using grab bar)
     and lift feet out of tub
   2) Stand up, using grab bar

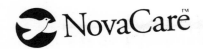 **NovaCare**™

<u>DISCHARGE SUMMARY</u>

Physical Therapy, (Occupational Therapy) Speech Therapy

Name: Diagnosis: IT Fx Neck   Date of Initial
                                    of Ⓛ Femur   Treatment: 1/3/89
Physician:
                               Treatment: Number of Treatments:
                                 self-care training
Facility: Boulder Manor   func. mobility trng.   Eval: 1
                                 therapeutic exercise   Part A 28
                                                            Part B 7

<u>History, Prior Level of Function:</u>
 Prior to hip fx pt. lived alone in Sr. Apt. complex. She was Ⓘ
in self-care, functional mobility. Three meals/day, laundry
a/ housekeeping services were provided. Pt. has supportive
family living close-by.

<u>Therapy Goals</u>	<u>Initial Status</u>	<u>Final Status</u> (Highest Level Reached)
1)↑ Ⓘ self-care		
grooming	mod Ⓐ	Ⓘ
oral care	min Ⓐ	Ⓘ
dressing	mod Ⓐ UⒺ; unable LⒺ	Ⓘ
toileting	max Ⓐ x 2	Ⓘ
bathing	not tested	min Ⓐ
2)↑ Ⓘ functional mobility		
bed mobility	max Ⓐ x 2	Ⓘ
transfers	max Ⓐ x 2	Ⓘ
w/c mobility	unable	Ⓘ
3)↑ Ⓑ UⒺ strength;	Grip strength Ⓡ 16# Ⓛ 14#	Ⓑ 20# Ⓛ 18#
ROM (shoulders)	60% active function	75% active function

Comments: Home visit/assessment completed 2/27/89. Pt. d/c'd home
c̄ following adapt. equip : raised toilet seat c̄ arms, tub grab bar,
tub safety bench, extended arm reacher, dressing stick, sock aid,
longhandled shoehorn, longhandled sponge.

Goals Met? Yes ✓   Partial_____   No_____

<u>Reason for Discharge:</u>
 Goals met ; pt d/c'd home 3/3/89

<u>Recommended Follow-up Care</u>
 1) Aide to Ⓐ c̄ bathing 3x/wk
 2) Pt. to follow UⒺ exercise program as per instructions

<u>3/3/89</u>   <u>O.T.</u>   _____OTR
Date of Discharge   Type of Therapy   Therapist Signature

NovaCare

PHYSICAL/OCCUPATIONAL/SPEECH THERAPY PROGRESS NOTES

NAME OF PATIENT _____   NAME OF FACILITY <u>Boulder Manor</u>

DATES	
1/3/89	O.T. eval completed as per physician's order. See data sheet for details. Medicare Rx completed ā sent to MD. Requested ā received telephone order for specific tx. Worked c̄ P.T. to present inservice to Nrsg. staff on transferring pt. bed ⇄ w/c. Pt. pleasant ā cooperative. Plan to begin tx 1/4/89. ⌐⌐⌐⌐⌐, OTR
1/4/89	Pt. seen in AM for self-care ā func. mobil. trng.; Ⓑ u/E therapeutic exercise. Instructed in grooming/oral care following set-up at sink; pt. required mod Ⓐ to comb hair, min Ⓐ to clean dentures, able to wash face/hands c̄ Ø Ⓐ. Following instruction in overhead technique, pt. able to doff blouse min Ⓐ; don mod Ⓐ. Ⓑ u/E therapeutic exercise: AROM x 10 (AAROM shoulders), cone stacking (11 on Ⓑ, 8 on Ⓛ). Xfer w/c → bed c̄ max Ⓐ x 2, toward Ⓡ, NWB Ⓛ u/E. Plan to cont tx 5x/wk as per eval goals. ⌐⌐⌐⌐, OTR
1/5/89	Pt. in bed; c/o Ⓛ hip pain. Instructed in bed mobility skills: rolled Ⓡ ā Ⓛ c̄ mod Ⓐ, scooted c̄ max Ⓐ. Xfer supine → sit max Ⓐ → w/c max Ⓐ x 2. Groomed following set-up at sink + min Ⓐ. Dressed u/E c̄ mod Ⓐ utilizing overhead tech. Xfer w/c ⇄ commode c̄ max Ⓐ x 2. Ⓑ u/E ther ex: AROM, AAROM x 10, cone stacking, balloon toss. Pt tolerated tx well. Cont 5x/wk. ⌐⌐⌐⌐, OTR
1/6/89	Pt. seen for self-care ā func. mobil. trng., ther. ex. Instructed in functional xfers for ADL's (w/c ⇄ commode; w/c ⇄ bed) c̄ pt. requiring mod/max Ⓐ x 2. Rolling in bed to ↑ ease in u/E dressing (Ⓛ min Ⓐ; Ⓡ mod Ⓐ). Undressed/dressed u/E c̄ min Ⓐ. Ⓑ u/E AROM + AAROM (shoulders) x 10. Pt. c/o fatigue, no additional ex. attempted. Attended weekly rehab. mtg. to discuss eval results, plan of tx. c̄ rehab team. Will schedule O.T. sessions in AM, as PT plans to see pt. in P.M. ⌐⌐⌐⌐, OTR

MONTH	1	2	3	4	5	6	7	8	9	10	11	12	13	14	15	16	17	18	19	20	21	22	23	24	25	26	27	28	29	30	31
JAN			E	X	X	X																									

P.T. _____	O.T. X	S.T. _____

page 2

NovaCare

PHYSICAL/OCCUPATIONAL/SPEECH THERAPY PROGRESS NOTES

NAME OF PATIENT _____ NAME OF FACILITY <u>Boulder Manor</u>

DATES	
WEEKLY SUMMARY	Pt. seen for eval + 3 tx sessions. Responding well to tx a beginning to show progress. Plan to cont tx 5x/wk as per eval goals. , OTR
1/9/89	Pt. seen for AM care trng; therap. ex. xfer supine + sit max Ⓐ → w/c mod/max Ⓐ x 2. Performed grooming/oral care c̄ min Ⓐ. Undressed/dressed u/e c̄ min Ⓐ + v.cues for technique. Began teaching pt. w/c mgmt. a w/c propulsion skills; following instructions + demonstration pt. required mod Ⓐ to propel 15'. ↓'d problem solving skills noted. , OTR
1/10/89	Pt. seen in AM. u/e dressing while supine in bed; required max Ⓐ. Pt. able to roll, but unable to bridge 2° obesity, weakness. xfer bed + w/c mod/max Ⓐ x 2. Dressed u/e c̄ min Ⓐ. Pt. required max Ⓐ to reposition self in w/c. Instructed in w/c mobility; propelled self 15' min/mod Ⓐ. Ⓑ u/e ther. ex: w/c push-ups x 10 (unable to lift buttocks), dowel ex: 2 sets x 11. Pt. motivated to be more Ⓘ; however expresses fear of pain upon any movement. , OTR
1/11/89	Pt. seen for self-care, func. mobil. trng, ther ex. Instructed in wt. shifts in w/c, trunk anterior flexion ex x 10 to ↑ sit → stand xfers. xfer w/c + commode c̄ max Ⓐ x 2. Pt. demonstrated ↓'d fear given ample time + opportunity to Ⓐ more in her xfer: "I feel more in control." Undressed/dressed u/e min Ⓐ. Ⓑ u/e dowel ex: 2 sets x 11. Pt. requested pain pill 2° Ⓛ hip pain: Nurse informed. ; OTR
1/12/89	Pt. seen for self-care a func. mobil. trng., ther ex. Undressed/dressed u/e min Ⓐ. Introduced use of adaptive equip. for u/e dressing. Instructed in techniques to don/doff shoes using extended arm reacher to open/close velcro tabs, long handled shoe horn. After 3 reps, pt. required

MONTH	1	2	3	4	5	6	7	8	9	10	11	12	13	14	15	16	17	18	19	20	21	22	23	24	25	26	27	28	29	30	31
JAN									X	X	X	X																			

P. T. _____	O. T. X	S. T. _____

page 2

NovaCare

PHYSICAL/OCCUPATIONAL/SPEECH THERAPY PROGRESS NOTES

NAME OF PATIENT _____ NAME OF FACILITY _Boulder Manor_

DATES	
1/12 cont.	max Ⓐ Ⓛ shoe, mod Ⓐ Ⓡ. Instructed in w/c mobility; pt. propelled self 25' c̄ min Ⓐ (in straight line). Plan to begin to work on maneuvering w/c about in room. , OTR
1/13/89	Pt. seen for self-care a func. mobility trng, u/e ther ex. xfer bed → w/c mod/max Ⓐ x1. Undressed/ dressed u/e occas. min Ⓐ; groomed c̄ set-up, occas. min Ⓐ. Instructed in w/c mgmt. skills (locking brakes, raising a swinging away legrests). Played "Balloon Volleyball" to ↑ active shoulder mvmt. No c/o ↑'d shoulder pain. Grip strength measured: 19 lbs Ⓡ 16 lbs Ⓛ. Attended weekly rehab mtg to discuss progress, goals c̄ rehab team. Pt. also c/o hip pain Ⓛ to P.T. , OTR
WEEKLY SUMMARY	Pt. progressing in all tx areas: u/e dressing from mod Ⓐ to min Ⓐ, w/c mobility from ll to mod Ⓐ; func. xfers max Ⓐ x2 to mod/max Ⓐ x2. Beginning to work on u/e dressing skills. Cont tx 5x/wk. OTR
1/16/89	Pt. seen in AM. Instructed 2 Nrsg. aides in w/c → commode xfers as pt. cont. to verbalize fear if a different person is involved in xfer. Anterior flexion ex x 10, wt. shifts in w/c prior to xfer. xfer w/c → commode c̄ max Ⓐ x1 + Ⓐ of another to pull pants up/down. Pt. performed grooming/oral care following set-up at sink. Don/doff shoes c̄ adapt. equip. + max Ⓐ Ⓛ, min/mod Ⓐ Ⓡ. Propelled w/c 50' c̄ min Ⓐ. , OTR
1/17/89 *14 day progress report sent to MD	Pt. seen for self-care trng c̄ instruction in use of adapt. equip, func. mobil. trng. a ther ex. Performed grooming/oral care Ⓘ at sink. Don/doff blouse occas. min Ⓐ. Following 3 reps + constant v. cues pt. able to don/doff Ⓡ shoe min Ⓐ; Ⓛ mod. Demonstrate use of dressing stick a dressing tape for donning pants.

MONTH	1	2	3	4	5	6	7	8	9	10	11	12	13	14	15	16	17	18	19	20	21	22	23	24	25	26	27	28	29	30	31
JAN													X			X	X														

P.T. _____ O.T. _X_ S.T. _____

NovaCare

PHYSICAL/OCCUPATIONAL/SPEECH THERAPY PROGRESS NOTES

NAME OF PATIENT _____ NAME OF FACILITY **Boulder Manor**

DATES	
1/17 cont.	but pt. stated she was too fatigued to try today. Anterior flexion, w/c push-ups × 10 to imp. sit ÷ stand xfer. Ⓑ u/e AROM × 10, cone stacking (13 on Ⓡ, 10 on Ⓛ). Cont tx. ⌒_____ OTR
1/18/89	Pt. seen in AM. Cheerful & cooperative. Dressed u/e c̄ v. cues + Ⓐ to hook bra. Recommended velcro closure on bras; pt will ask daughter to sew them on. Don/doff shoes c̄ use of adapt. equip: mod Ⓐ Ⓛ, Ⓘ Ⓡ. Instructed new nurse's aide in w/c ⇄ commoc xfer. Required max Ⓐ of 1 + Ⓐ of another to pull pants up/down. xfer w/c ÷ bed max Ⓐ of 1 + SBA of 1. Instructed in rolling, scooting, bridging skills to pull pants up/down: required mod Ⓐ. Ⓑ u/e AROM exercises c̄ dowel (each joint × 10) while supine in bed, no c/o pain in shoulders. Pt. displayinc v̄'d fear, ↑'d active participation in functional mobility. Cont tx 5×/wk. ⌒_____ OTR
1/19/89	Pt. seen in A.M. In good spirits; daughter present to observe session. Introduced use of dressing stick for l/e dressing & demonstrated its use. Pt. required mod/max Ⓐ to get slacks over feet, then remove them. Instructed in sit ⇄ stand xfers to ↑ ease for l/e dressing (× 5) c̄ pt. requiring v. cues for correct position & NWB status Ⓛ l/e + mod Ⓐ. Don/doff blouse c̄ v. cues + Ⓐ to hook bra. Daughter will bring bras c̄ velcro closures next week. Ⓑ u/e AROM × 10, cone stacking (14 on Ⓡ, 11 on Ⓛ), balloor toss. No c/o shoulder pain. Cont tx. ⌒_____ OTR
1/20/89	Pt seen for self-care & func. mobil. trng. ther ex. Instructed in use of adapt. equip for l/e dressing. Using dressing stick, pt able to don/doff panties min/mod Ⓐ; slacks mod Ⓐ (excluding standing to pull them up). Don/doff Ⓡ shoe Ⓘ, Ⓛ shoe min/mod Ⓐ

MONTH	1	2	3	4	5	6	7	8	9	10	11	12	13	14	15	16	17	18	19	20	21	22	23	24	25	26	27	28	29	30	31
JAN																		X	X	X											

P. T. _____	O. T. __X__	S. T. _____

page 2

NovaCare

PHYSICAL/OCCUPATIONAL/SPEECH THERAPY PROGRESS NOTES

NAME OF PATIENT _____ NAME OF FACILITY <u>Boulder Manor</u>

DATES	
1/20 cont.	Undressed/dressed U/E c̄ (A) to hook bra. Pt. propelled w/c 100' c̄ min (A). Sit ⇄ stand xfers x 5 c̄ mod (A). (B) U/E ther ex AROM x 10, bean bag toss. Pt. stated she enjoyed bean bag toss. Pt. is displaying mild problem solving skills in all ADL skills a̅ needs frequent verbal cueing. Attended weekly rehab mtg. to discuss pt's case c̄ Rehab team. r_____, OTR
WEEKLY SUMMARY	Pt. cont. to make progress in all tx areas: U/E dressing from min (A) to (A) to hook bra only, L/E from max to mod (A), grooming/oral care from set-up, occas. min (A) to (I), func. xfers from mod/max (A) x 2 to max (A) x 1 + SBA of 1. w/c mobility skills ↑ from mod (A) to min (A) 100'. Plan to cont tx 5x/wk as per stated goals. r_____, OTR
1/23/89	Pt. seen in AM for self-care a̅ func. mobil. trng, ther ex. Pt's daughter had brought in bras c̄ velcro closures. Instructed in donning/doffing bra x 3; on 3rd attempt pt was (I). L/E dressing c̄ use of adapt. equip. Min/mod (A) to don/doff panties a̅ slacks (s̄ standing to pull them up). Don/doff shoes x 2 c̄ adapt equip + min (A) (L). Pt. refused any further tx "I feel like I'm coming down c̄ something." Nrsg. informed. r_____, OTR
1/24/89	Attempted to see pt in AM. Stated she wasn't feeling well. Checked c̄ Nrsg; pt had temp. of 100.7°; "flu-like" symptoms. No tx. r_____, OTR
1/25/89	Pt. ill. No tx r_____, OTR
1/26/89	Pt. ill No tx. r_____, OTR
1/27/89	Pt. seen in AM. Stated she was feeling better a̅ ready to resume tx. Cleared c̄ Nrsg. Instructed in dressing skills c̄ use of adapt. equip. Undressed/dressed U/E c̄ v. cues. Don/doff L/E clothing (s̄ coming to stand)

MONTH	1	2	3	4	5	6	7	8	9	10	11	12	13	14	15	16	17	18	19	20	21	22	23	24	25	26	27	28	29	30	31
																							X	I	I	I	X				

P. T. _____   O. T. X   S. T. _____

page 2

Case B (continued)

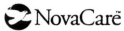NovaCare

PHYSICAL/OCCUPATIONAL/SPEECH THERAPY PROGRESS NOTES

NAME OF FACILITY _Boulder Manor_____

NAME OF PATIENT _____

DATES	
1/27 cont.	c̄ min Ⓐ. Worked on sit ⇄ stand xfers in preparation for standing to pull pants up. Required min/mod Ⓐ; able to let go c̄ 1 hand. Expressed ↓'d fear, no c/o Ⓛ hip pain. Ⓑ u/e AROM x 10, cone stacking (13 on Ⓡ 11 on Ⓛ). Pt. fatigued easily, but no notable func. loss following bout c̄ "flu." Attended weekly rehab. mtg. to discuss pt's case c̄ rehab team. P.T. reports Pt. to have x-ray 2/1/89 c̄ possible change in weight-bearing status on that date. ⌐⌐⌐⌐⌐, OTR
WEEKLY SUMMARY	Pt. ill 3 days this week. Progressed from mod Ⓐ to min/mod Ⓐ sit ⇄ stand xfers. Expressing ↓'d fear when standing, & now able to let go of walker c̄ 1 hand. Pt now Ⓘ in u/e dressing c̄ use of velcro-closure bras. Cont tx 5x/wk. ⌐⌐⌐⌐⌐, OTR
1/30/89	Pt. seen for self-care & func. mobil. trng, ther ex. Dressed u/e Ⓘ. Dressed L/e c̄ instruction in use of adapt. equip + min Ⓐ. Sit ⇄ stand xfers x 5 c̄ min Ⓐ (NWB Ⓛ L/e). Pt. able to adjust her position in chair c̄ min Ⓐ when uncomfortable. Propelled w/c 100' Ⓘ incl. maneuvering doorway; demon-strating imp. problem-solving skills. Ⓑ u/e ex incl. dowel ex. 2 sets x 10 + bean bag toss. Plan to begin working on pulling pants up/down. ⌐⌐⌐⌐⌐, OTR
1/31/89	Pt. seen in AM. Instructed in L/e dressing c̄ use of adapt. equip. Dressed L/e (excl. Ted hose) c̄ min Ⓐ + mod/max Ⓐ to pull pants up/down. xfer w/c ⇄ commode mod/max Ⓐ x 1. Pt. propelled w/c 150' Ⓘ today (distance to dining room). Ⓑ u/e ther ex incl. Balloon volleyball, bean bag toss, dowel ex x 12. Informed Nrsg. of pt's ability to propel w/c to d.r. They will encourage her to propel herself at least 2 meals/day. ⌐⌐⌐⌐⌐, OTR

MONTH	1	2	3	4	5	6	7	8	9	10	11	12	13	14	15	16	17	18	19	20	21	22	23	24	25	26	27	28	29	30	31
																														X	X

P.T. _____   O.T. _X_   S.T. _____

page 2

NovaCare

PHYSICAL/OCCUPATIONAL/SPEECH THERAPY PROGRESS NOTES

NAME OF PATIENT _____ NAME OF FACILITY __Boulder Manor__

DATES	
2/1/89	Pt. at Dr's Appt. this AM, so seen by O.T. in early P.M. X-ray reveals fx healing well; pt now PWB (L) U/E. Instructed in U/E dressing skills: pt. required occas. min (A) (L) shoe, min/SBA to come to stand, mod (A) to pull pants up/down. xfer w/c ⇄ commode c̄ mod (A). Pt. refused U/E ther ex as she still had to go to PT a didn't want to be too tired. Plan to observe pt's ambulation skills c̄ P.T. 2/2. ~ _____, OTR
2/2/89	Pt. seen in AM for self-care a func. mobil. trng,
*Medicare	U/E ther ex. Undressed/dressed U/E (I); U/E c̄
re-cert	mod (A) to pull pants up/down (PWB (L) U/E). M.D.
sent to	d/c'd order for Ted hose, so demonstrated use
MD	of sock aid to pt. for donning socks. (B) U/E ther ex AROM x 11 (each joint), cone stacking (14 on (R), 12 on (L)). Grip strength measured: 20#'s (R), 17# (L). Observed ambulation skills c̄ PT; requires walker + min/mod (A). Plan to begin ambulating pt. to bathroom for toilet xfers. ~ _____, OTR
2/3/89	Pt. seen for self-care a func. mobil. trng, U/E ther ex. Undressed/dressed c̄ adapt. equip + mod (A) to pull pants up/down. Instructed in use of sock aid. Following 3 reps, pt was able to don socks c̄ occas. min (A); doff socks using dressing stick (I) (R), min (A) (L). Ambulated 18' via walker (PWB (L) U/E) a toileted (incl. xfer; pulling pants up/down) c̄ min/mod (A). (B) U/E ther ex: dowel ex: 2 sets x 12, Balloon volleyball. Attended weekly rehab mtg. to discuss pt's progress c̄ Rehab team. Nsg. reports pt. is propelling self to dining room 2 meals/day. ~ _____, OTR
WEEKLY	Pt. has made significant progress this week. U/E dressing
SUMMARY	imp. from mod (A) to min (A). Pt is now able to ambulat

MONTH	1	2	3	4	5	6	7	8	9	10	11	12	13	14	15	16	17	18	19	20	21	22	23	24	25	26	27	28	29	30	31
FEB	X	X	X																												

P. T. _____	O. T. _X_	S. T. _____

page 2

● NovaCare™

PHYSICAL/OCCUPATIONAL/SPEECH THERAPY PROGRESS NOTES

NAME OF PATIENT _____   NAME OF FACILITY <u>Boulder Manor</u>

DATES	
WEEKLY SUMMARY, cont.	to bathroom via walker (PWB (L)U/E) a/ toilet c̄ min/ mod Ⓐ (imp. from mod Ⓐ.). W/c mobility has imp. from min Ⓐ to Ⓘ a/ pt. now propels self to meals. Cont tx 5x/wk. ⌐ _____ , OTR
2/6/89	Pt seen in AM. Pt. lying in bed. ℅ stiffness Ⓑ shoulders. U/E AROM (each joint x 12). Xfer supine→sit mod A → w/c min/mod Ⓐ. Dressed U/E Ⓘ; L/E c̄ occas. min Ⓐ + mod Ⓐ for standing balance while pulling up pants. Ambulated to bathroom a/ toileted c̄ min/mod Ⓐ. Raised toilet seat in place, but grab bar appears to strain shoulder. Will request raised seat c̄ arms to ↑ ease of xfer, ↓ strain on shoulder. Pt. stated "I finally feel like I'll be able to get well enough to go home." Cont tx 5x/wk. ⌐ _____ ,OTR
2/7/89	Pt seen in AM. Ⓑ U/E AROM x 12. Goniometric measurements taken Ⓑ shoulders. Ⓡ: flexion 130°, abduction 125°, adduction 110°, IR 60°, ER 60°. Ⓛ flexion 110°, abduction 110°, adduction 100°, IR 60°, ER 65°. Measurements show an average ↑ of 10° each movement. No ℅ shoulder pain. Instructed in L/E dressing techniques c̄ use of adaptive equipment (sock aid, dressing stick, reacher, long handled shoehorn). Pt. required v. cues, occas. min Ⓐ to manipulate equip. + mod Ⓐ for standing balance/pulling pants up. Raised toilet seat c̄ arms in place. Pt xferred to/from toilet c̄ min Ⓐ. Pt stated new seat was much easier. ⌐ _____ OTR
2/8/89	Pt. seen in AM for self-care a/ func mobil. trng, ther ex. Xfer supine→sit → w/c min/mod Ⓐ. Dressed c̄ occas. min Ⓐ + adapt. equip. + min/mod Ⓐ standing/pulling pants up. Pt. has difficulty

MONTH	1	2	3	4	5	6	7	8	9	10	11	12	13	14	15	16	17	18	19	20	21	22	23	24	25	26	27	28	29	30	31
FEB						X	X	X																							

P. T. _____	O. T. ╳	S. T. _____

page 2

NovaCare

PHYSICAL/OCCUPATIONAL/SPEECH THERAPY PROGRESS NOTES

NAME OF PATIENT _____   NAME OF FACILITY __Boulder Manor__

DATES	
2/8 cont.	Pulling pants up in back 2° obesity. Ambulated to b.r. via walker ā toileted c̄ min/mod Ⓐ. Ⓑ U/E ex: cone stacking (15 on Ⓡ, 12 on Ⓛ), bean bag toss. Cont tx 5x/wk. ⌒ ~~~~~~~, OTR
2/9/89	Pt. seen in AM for self-care, func. mobil trng, ther ex. Undressed/dressed c̄ v. cues + Ⓐ for standing balance. Quizzed pt. re sequence for dressing ā stressed its importance r/t energy conservation ā safety factors. Ambulated to b.r. ā toileted c̄ min Ⓐ. Ⓑ U/E dowel ex: 2 sets × 13. Plan to cont tx toward ↑ing func. Ⓘ. ⌒ ~~~~~~~, OTR
2/10/89	Pt. seen in AM. Worked on ↑ing standing endurance. Pt. stood c̄ walker at sink ā completed grooming, oral care, hygiene tasks. Pt needed to stop ×2 to sit ā rest. Undressed/ dressed c̄ occas min Ⓐ using adapt. equip + min Ⓐ for standing balance. Ⓑ U/E ex: bean bag toss, dowel ex × 13. Attended weekly rehab. mtg to discuss case c̄ Rehab team. U.R. Subcommittee denial given. Plan to cont. tx 5x/wk for 1 wk, then 3x/wk (Part B) for 2 wks. ⌒ ~~~~~~~, OTR
WEEKLY SUMMARY	Pt. cont. to progress in all tx areas: U/E dressing from min Ⓐ to occas. min Ⓐ; toileting from min/mod Ⓐ to min Ⓐ. Ⓑ U/E shoulder movements have ↑'d approx 10° each movement. ⌒ ~~~~ ⌐ C
2/13/89	Pt. seen in AM. Undressed/dressed c̄ adapt equip + min Ⓐ to stand ā pull up pants. Pt. demonstrating imp. standing balance; no longer voices fear of falling. Quizzed pt × 3 re dressing sequence; 75% accurate. Instructed in func. mobil. skills: standing at

MONTH	1	2	3	4	5	6	7	8	9	10	11	12	13	14	15	16	17	18	19	20	21	22	23	24	25	26	27	28	29	30	31
FEB									X	X			X																		

P.T. _____   O.T. _X_   S.T. _____

NovaCare

PHYSICAL/OCCUPATIONAL/SPEECH THERAPY PROGRESS NOTES

NAME OF PATIENT _____   NAME OF FACILITY Boulder Manor

DATES	
	walker a/ opening a/ closing door, closet, drawers. Pt. required v. cues r/t safety. Ⓑ U/E ex: wall pulleys ½# wt : 2 sets x 12. ⌐ ,OTR
2/14/89	Pt. seen in AM. xfer supine → sit → w/c min Ⓐ. Dressed c̄ 80% accuracy for sequencing skills (energy conservation, safety); required min Ⓐ to stand a/ pull up pants. Ambulated via walker to bathroom (PWB Ⓛ U/E) a/ toileted c̄ contact guard Ⓐ for xfer, min Ⓐ to pull pants up. Ⓑ U/E ex: wall pulleys ½# wt: 2 sets x 12. Cont tx. ⌐ ,OTR
2/15/89	Pt. refused tx 2° diarrhea. ⌐ ,OTR
2/16/89	Pt. seen in AM. xfer supine → sit min Ⓐ → w/c contact guard Ⓐ. Dressed c̄ 80% accuracy for sequencing; min Ⓐ to stand a/ pull up pants. Stood at sink to perform grooming/ hygiene tasks c̄ contact guard Ⓐ. Ⓑ U/E ex: cone stacking (16 on Ⓡ, 14 on Ⓛ). Grip strength measured: 20# Ⓡ, 18# Ⓛ. Plan to begin seeing pt. 3x/wk (Part B benefits). Phone conf. c̄ daughter to discuss new tx schedule, set up appt. for home assessment. ⌐ ,OTR
2/17/89	Pt. seen for self-care a/ func. mobil. trng; ther ex. undressed/dressed using adapt equip + min Ⓐ to stand a/ pull up pants. Groomed while standing at sink c̄ contact guard Ⓐ * 1 rst break. Ambulated to b.r. a/ toileted c̄ contact guard/min Ⓐ. Ⓑ U/E ex: balloon volleyball, dowel ex: 2 sets x 13. Attended weekly rehab mtg. to discuss pt's case c̄ rehab team. Plan to begin working on tub xfer trng. ⌐ ,OTR
WEEKLY SUMMARY	Progress this week as follows: U/E dressing from occas. min Ⓐ to Ⓐ for standing balance only, while

MONTH	1	2	3	4	5	6	7	8	9	10	11	12	13	14	15	16	17	18	19	20	21	22	23	24	25	26	27	28	29	30	31
FEB														X	I	X	X														

P.T. _____	O.T. __X__	S.T. _____

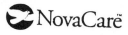 NovaCare

PHYSICAL/OCCUPATIONAL/SPEECH THERAPY PROGRESS NOTES

NAME OF PATIENT _____ NAME OF FACILITY __Boulder Manor__

DATES	
WEEKLY SUMMARY, cont.	Pulling up pants. Toilet xfer imp. from min Ⓐ to contact guard Ⓐ. Pt. now able to stand at sink for grooming tasks demonstrating ↑'d endurance + balance. Plan to cont tx 3x/wk for 2 wks to further ↑ Ⓘ for d/c home.
2/20/89	Pt. seen for tub xfer / bathing trng. Demonstrated safe tub xfer x 2 using tub grab bar + tub safety bench. Pt xfer to/from tub c̄ mod Ⓐ to lift Ⓛ leg. Bathed using long handled sponge c̄ occas. min Ⓐ. Phone conf. c̄ daughter to recommend getting raised toilet seat c̄ arms, tub grab bar, & tub safety bench. Home visit planned for 2/27. Received t.o. from M.D. for home assessment. _____, OTR
2/22/89	Pt. lying in bed. xfer supine → sit occas. min Ⓐ → w/c SBA. Dressed c̄ SBA + v. cues for sequencing. Pt. given written instructions for correct sequence during undressing/dressing. Copy placed in chart. When pt. gets out of sequence she has poor problem solving skills & becomes nervous. Pt. amb. via walker to b.r. & toilet c̄ SBA. Adheres to PWB status Ⓛ LE. Ⓑ U/E ther ex: cone stacking (17 on Ⓡ, 15 on Ⓛ), bean bag toss. _____, OTR
2/24/89	Pt. seen for dressing / bathing trng. Undressed (using written sequence instructions) c̄ SBA + use of adapt. equip. Pt. xfer in/out of tub c̄ min/mod Ⓐ to lift Ⓛ leg (using tub bench, grab bar). Bathed, dried self c̄ occas. min Ⓐ + use of long handled sponge. Dressed c̄ SBA. Attended weekly rehab. mtg. to discuss pt. c̄ team. Recommend pt. have aide to help her c̄ bathing at home. Social Worker will contact daughter to make arrangements. _____, OTR

MONTH	1	2	3	4	5	6	7	8	9	10	11	12	13	14	15	16	17	18	19	20	21	22	23	24	25	26	27	28	29	30	31
FEB																				X		X		X							

P. T. _____ O. T. __X__ S. T. _____

page 2

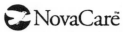

NovaCare

PHYSICAL/OCCUPATIONAL/SPEECH THERAPY PROGRESS NOTES

NAME OF PATIENT _____   NAME OF FACILITY __Boulder Manor__

DATES	
WEEKLY SUMMARY	Pt. cont. to make progress toward d/c home. 4° dressing has imp. from Ⓐ for standing balance + v. cues to SBA; toileting from contact guard to SBA. Began working on bathing skills; pt. requires min Ⓐ ᵃ will need aide to Ⓐ her at home for safety reasons. Plan to cont tx 3x/wk. for 1 wk c̄ home assessment. Scheduled 2/27. ⌐⌐⌐⌐⌐⌐⌐⌐, OTR
2/27/89	Pt. seen for home visit/assessment. Pt's daughter present. Pt. xfer into car c̄ min Ⓐ Ⓛ4°. Amb. up sidewalk at home c̄ SBA. Ø stairs at home. Throw rugs removed from floors for safety reasons. Bedroom: pt xfer in/out of bed c̄ v. cues. Able to manage doors ᵃ drawers s̄ difficulty. Arranged clothes in top drawers. Living Area: furniture re-arranged slightly to ↑ ease of maneuvering walker. Pt. able to get into/out of all chairs ᵃ on/off sofa Ⓘ. Bathroom: tub grab bar + tub safety bench in place. Bath aide services set up for 3x/wk. Raised toilet seat c̄ arms in place. Pt. xfer c̄ supervision. Kitchen: sm refrigerator, sink only. Pt. receives 3 meals/day in common dining room. Pt amb. c̄ supervision only to d.r. Saw several friends ᵃ informed them of return home at end of week. Returned to SNF ᵃ held conf. c̄ Nrsg, PT, Soc. Worker re results of home visit. Plan to cont tx 2 more sessions to further ↑ Ⓘ for d/c home. ⌐⌐⌐⌐⌐⌐⌐⌐, OTR

MONTH	1	2	3	4	5	6	7	8	9	10	11	12	13	14	15	16	17	18	19	20	21	22	23	24	25	26	27	28	29	30	31
FEB																											X				

P. T. _____	O. T. __X__	S. T. _____

page 2

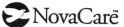 NovaCare

PHYSICAL/OCCUPATIONAL/SPEECH THERAPY PROGRESS NOTES

NAME OF PATIENT _____ NAME OF FACILITY Boulder Manor

DATES	
3/1/89	Pt. seen in AM for self-care a/ func. mobil. trng., ther ex. xfer supine in bed → chair c̄ supervision. Amb. via walker to sink a/ performed grooming /oral care while standing at sink; did not require any rest periods. Pt dressed c̄ supervision + adapt equip. Referred to dressing sequence instructions x 2, but did not require V. cues. Toileted c̄ supervision. (B) u/e AROM ex x 12. Goniometric measurements taken (B) shoulders. (R): flexion 130°, abduction 130°, adduction 110°, IR 60°, ER 70° (L): flexion 120°, abduction 115°, adduction 110°, IR 60°, ER 70° Measurements show an average ↑ of 15° each movement. Plan to see pt. for final tx session 3/3/89. N̶i̶_____, OTR
3/3/89	Pt. seen for final tx session. Able to complete AM care routine (I) c̄ use of adapt. equip (bed mobility, xfers, dressing, grooming, toileting). Daughter present to (A) c̄ d/c. Pt. provided c̄ following adaptive equip: reacher, dressing stick, sock aid, long handled shoehorn, long handled sponge. Also given written instructions for dressing sequence, u/e AROM exercises, bathtub xfers. Grip strength measurements taken: 20# (R), 18# (L). Pt. to be d/c'd home to apt. this date c̄ (A) for bathing 3x/wk. D/C summary completed a/ sent to MD. N̶i̶_____ ____, OTR

MONTH	1	2	3	4	5	6	7	8	9	10	11	12	13	14	15	16	17	18	19	20	21	22	23	24	25	26	27	28	29	30	31
MARCH	X		X	D/C																											

P. T. _____	O. T. X	S. T. _____

page 2

PATIENT DATA SHEET

FUNCTIONAL DIAGNOSIS: _ℓ CVA, ℛ Hemi, global aphasia_

REFERRING PHYSICIAN (NRH): _OZER_
REASON FOR REFERRAL: _Comprehensive Rehab._

HISTORY:
  Date of onset: _9-5-89_
  Description of Condition: _Admitted to N. Va Dr's Hosp 9/5 c̄ sudden HA, ℛ sided weakness, unresponsive - admitted to NORH 9/28 - receive PT, OT, SLP. CT reveals intracerebral hemorrhage ℓ fronto-parietal c̄ compression of lateral ventrical._
  Previous Therapy/Surgery/Dates: _∅_

Other PMHX: _HYPOTENSION, HX DEPRESSION c̄ HYPOTHYROID CONDITION. Orthostatic hypotension, hypokalcemia_

FAMILY/ENVIRONMENTAL HISTORY: S Ⓜ W D _LIVES c̄ WIFE, SON + DTR. IN-LAW, GRAND CHILD IN HOUSE - HOUSE IS ONE LEVEL c̄ 5 STEPS TO ENTER._

ORIENTATION: _UNABLE TO ASSESS 2' TO GLOBAL APHASIA._

OCCUPATION: _RETIRED REAL ESTATE BROKER / ENGINEER, enjoyed gardening, carpentry, mechanical tasks, music, reading, game shows, homemaking tasks_
DOMINANCE: Left (Right) Ambidextrous
SUBJECTIVE INFORMATION:
  Complaints: _Pt expresses frustration over inability to communicate + to complete simple tasks._

  Priorities: _FAMILY GOALS: "HELP HIMSELF MORE, BE AMBULATORY, CONTINENT"_

  Activity Level: _prior to 1987 - very active, employed, since 1987 - depressed, unemployed, inactive_

  Assistive devices used: _has rental wc, glasses_

PROBABLE DISCHARGE DISPOSITION: _HOME c̄ FAMILY IF POSSIBLE._

Therapist(s):   Date: _10/27/89_

NAME   INITIAL

NRH
NATIONAL
REHABILITATION
HOSPITAL
THERAPY SERVICES
FORM 200/210-008   10/85

PATIENT DATA SHEET

ADDITIONAL OBJECTIVE DATA

Address appropriate categories(s) from the following: Skin status, Respiratory Status, Muscle Tone, Balance, Coordination, Endurance, Posture/Body Mechanics, Gait, Reflex Testing, Reflex Integration, Prosthetics/Orthotics, Musculoskeletal Assessment, Cognitive/Behavioral Status.

10/27/89 Ⓡ scapula demonstrates "winging" from chest wall. Ⓡ Scapula is elevated and abducted on chest wall. Ⓡ UE appears ∅ to have no AROM, however this is difficult to assess 2° pt's ↓ ability to follow commands. PROM WFL c̄ Mod ↑'d tone at shoulder, elbow, wrist + hand. Mild edema present in Ⓡ hand. There is 1½ finger subluxation at Ⓡ shoulder.

10/30/89 In gravity eliminated position, pt demonstrates active elbow flexion & extension & horizonal abduction within synergy. Severe tightness noted upon PROM of pecs & forearm ~~error~~ pronators. Moderate tightness noted in upper traps & wrist/finger flexors. Active movement is limited by tone and by pt's inability to follow commands.

11/2/89 Physical Therapy

<u>Gait</u>: Ambulation c̄ WBQC attempted. Pt. required mod Ⓐ ⇒ max Ⓐ to ambulate x 5'. Gait deviations include: ① inconsistent c̄ ability to advance Ⓡ LE in sequence c̄ v. cues ② ↓'d isolated movement c̄ swing (i.e. leg advanced c̄ hip & knee flexion/ abduction synergy. Pt. able to shift ᶜ⁽¹⁰⁻²⁰%⁾ᴰ wt. Ⓔ in stance. Pt. requiring manual Ⓐ to advance cane in sequence. Stairs not tested.

<u>Balance</u>: maintains sitting unsupported through mod. excursion, maintains standing x ▓▓▓▓▓▓▓▓ requires min → mod Ⓘ to achieve symmetry & Ⓡ LE extension

DATE 11/1/89

DIAGNOSIS (L) CVA, global aphasia

SENSORY EVALUATION

PAIN: SHARP/DULL

COMMENTS: _Unable to assess 2°_
aphasia - pt appears to experie
(R)UE pain at shoulder, forearm &
wrist during PROM exercises (cm)
Unable to assess 2° un-
reliability of pr. responses

VIBRATION: (256 cps)

Indicate most intact distal bony prominence. Test distal to
proximal in the following order:

UE	LE
DIP INDEX FINGER	GREAT TOE
WRIST	ANKLE
ELBOW	KNEE
CLAVICLE	ILIAC CREST

COMMENTS: _Unable to assess 2° aphas_
NT in LE 2° cognitive
deficits

NRH

N A T I O N A L
R E H A B I L I T A T I O N
H O S P I T A L

**THERAPY
SERVICES**

KEY:

NORMAL:	□
ABSENT:	■
DECREASED:	↓
HYPERSENSITIVE:	↑
NOT TESTED	NT

DOUBLE SIMULTANEOUS STIMULATION

HANDS	KEY: (CHECK)	FEET
NT	NORMAL: EXTINGUISHES NEITHER	NT
	EXTINGUISHES R (WHEN BOTH TOUCHED)	
↓	EXTINGUISHES L (WHEN BOTH TOUCHED)	↓

STEREOGNOSIS

Occlude patient's vision. Manipulate objects in hand if patient is unable to do so. + = correct response; − = incorrect (explain)

R	OBJECT	L
NT	SAFETY PIN	NT
	COIN	
	SCREW	
	NAIL	
	BUTTON	
↓	KEY	↓

R	SHAPE	L
NT	CIRCLE	NT
	TRIANGLE	
↓	SQUARE	↓

PROPRIOCEPTION: Position Sense

a. Motion: Difference between up and down by passively moving upper extremity, holding at bony prominences.

RUE		LUE
NT	SHOULDER	NT
	ELBOW	
	WRIST	
	THUMB	
	INDEX FINGER	
↓	LITTLE FINGER	↓

RLE		LLE
NT	HIP	NT
	KNEE	
	ANKLE	
↓	TOES	↓

b. Position: Patient duplicates position of moved side with other side.

RUE		LUE
NT	SHOULDER	NT
	ELBOW	
	WRIST	
	THUMB	
	INDEX FINGER	
↓	LITTLE FINGER	↓

RLE		LLE
NT	HIP	NT
	KNEE	
	ANKLE	
↓	TOES	↓

KEY: NORMAL: N
IMPAIRED: I
ABSENT: O
NOT TESTED: NT

NT = Not tested as results are unreliable 2° communication deficits CVA

THERAPY SERVICES
RANGE OF MOTION

PT ☐ OT ☐

00-40-95

LEFT							RIGHT			
PROM	AROM	PROM	AROM				PROM	AROM	PROM	AROM
		10-27	10-27		DATE		10-27	10-27		
		cm	cm		EXAMINER'S INITIALS		cm	cm		
		WFL	WFL	S H O U L D E R	FLEXION 0 - 180	S H O U L D E R	0-130°	X		
					EXTENSION 0 - 60					
					ABDUCTION 0 - 180		0-119°			
					ADDUCTION 180 - 0		119-0°			
					HORIZONTAL ABDUCTION 0 - 90		0-90°			
					HORIZONTAL ADDUCTION 0 - 45		0-45°			
					INTERNAL ROTATION 0 - 90					
					EXTERNAL ROTATION 0 - 90					
				ELBOW	FLEXION 0 - 150	ELBOW	0-150°			
					EXTENSION 150 - 0		150-0°			
				FORE ARM	SUPINATION 0 - 90	FORE ARM	0°			
					PRONATION 0 - 90		0-90°			
				W R I S T	FLEXION 0 - 90	W R I S T	0-88°			
					EXTENSION 0 - 70		0-45°			
					RADIAL DEVIATION 0 - 20		0-12°			
					ULNAR DEVIATION 0 - 30		0-25°			
				T H U M B	MP FLEXION 0 - 70	T H U M B	0-60°			
					MP EXTENSION 70 - 0		60-0°			
					IP FLEXION 0 - 90		0-60°			
					IP EXTENSION 90 - 0		60-0°			
					WEB SPAN (distal crease to edge of IP joint thumb in palmar abduction		NT			
					ADDUCTION 50 - 0					
					OPPOSITION TO _____ FINGER					
					OPPOSITION (=cm)					

EXTENSION/FLEXION

PROM	AROM	PROM	AROM				PROM	AROM	PROM	AROM
				F I N G E R S	2 90 - 0 MCP 0 - 90 2	F I N G E R S	0-90			
					3 3		0-90			
					4 4		0-90			
					5 5		0-90			
					2 120 - 0 PIP 0 - 120 2		0-110°			
					3 3		0-106°			
					4 4		0-105°			
					5 5		0-105°			
					2 90 - 0 DIP 0 - 90 2		0-46°			
					3 3		0-46°			
					4 4		0-80°			
					5 5		0-60°			
					2 FLEXION TO DPC 2		NT			
					3 3					
					4 4					
					5 5					

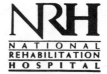

THERAPY SERVICES
RANGE OF MOTION

								RIGHT			
PROM	AROM	PROM	AROM					PROM	AROM	PROM	AROM
		10/30	10/30		DATE			10/30	10/30		
		cms	cms		EXAMINER'S INITIALS			cms	cms		
		WFL	WFL	H I P	FLEXION 0 - 125	H I P		WFL	*		
					EXTENSION 0 - 15						
					ABDUCTION 0 - 45						
					ADDUCTION 45 - 0						
					INTERNAL ROTATION 0 - 45						
					EXTERNAL ROTATION 0 - 45						
				KNEE	FLEXION 0 - 135	KNEE		WFL			
					EXTENSION 135 - 0						
				ANKLE	DORSIFLEXION 0 - 10	ANKLE		WFL			
					PLANTARFLEXION 0 - 45						
				FORE FOOT	INVERSION 0 - 30	FORE FOOT					
					EVERSION 0 - 15						

EXTENSION/FLEXION

					1	MTP	1		WFL	∅		
					2		2					
					3		3					
					4		4					
				T O E S	5		5	T O E S				
					1	IP	1					
					2		2					
					3		3					
					4		4					
					5		5					

COMMENTS: 10/2? ① LE AROM WFL - pt exhibits difficulty following motor commands or demonstration of AROM. (cms)
pt often tried to grab therapists hand when asked to perform a movement (cms)

* pt. moving in synergy ® LE: ® hip √ c̄ abduction/ext. rotation; ® knee √ accompanied c̄ ® hip ext. rotation; in supine ® ankle dorsiflexion only c̄ knee & hip √; hip ext. rotation thru ⅓ ROM; hip int. rotation trace

X see back of pt. data sheet for report of active ® LE mov't.

THERAPIST(S):

Name	Initials
Name	Initials

DLS / FUNCTIONAL PERFORMANCE

Dx: ① CVA, global aphasia   Dominance: ⓇR

OT ☒   PT ☐

KEY:
1—Independent without equipment
2—Independent with equipment
3—Independent with set-up
4—Supervision
5—Assistance
6—Dependent

EATING	Date	11-2		
	Initials	CM		
open containers		6	-	
cut meat		NT		
butter bread		NT		
eat with fork		4		
eat with spoon		4		
drink from glass		4		
finger feed		4		
maneuver utensils		4		
oral motor function		4		

comments: Required cues for proper use of utensils, use of straw & rate of eating (CM)

HYGIENE & GROOMING	Date	10-31		
	Initials	CM		
wash hands cues for Ⓡ hand		4		
wash face		4		
brush teeth		NT		
clean dentures		NT		
comb hair cues for proper use of comb		4		
wash hair		NT		
set hair		NA		
apply make-up		NA		
shave—elec. & safety		NT		
deodorant		NT		
trim & clean nails		NT		
manage wig/toupe		NA		
manage glasses/contacts		NT		

comments:

BATHING	Date	10-31		
	Initials	CM		
shower c̄ shower chair Mod		5		
tub		NT		
sponge bath		NT		

comments: (equipment) Required demonstration, Mod physical assist + cues to attend to Ⓑ LE/Ⓡ LE (CM)

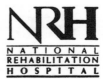

DRESSING (on/off)	Date	10-31				
	Initials	CM				
		O	F	O	F	O	F
hospital clothing	Max		5			
bra/male support		N	A			
undershirt, T-shirt	Max	5	5			
button front blouse/shirt	Max	5				
panties/shorts		N	A			
slacks	Max	5				
skirt/slip		N	A			
dress		N	A			
socks, hose	Mod/Max	5	5			
shoes	Mod/Max	5				
braces		N	A			
sweater		N	T			
coat						
boots						
gloves/mittens						
scarf						
tie						
other						

comments: Pt required much cueing + demonstr. 2° difficulty following commands. ↓ demonstrated neglect of Ⓑ LE/Ⓡ LE & difficulty distinguishing Ⓡ from Ⓛ extremities. Misuse of objects noted (CM)

TOILETING	Date	10-31		
	Initials	CM		
bath use appro. reg. or adapted		NT		
total bath care				
bed pan				
urinal				
empty catheter				
apply int. catheter				
skin inspection				
sterilization				
tampax				
suppository				
dig stim.				

comments:

NRH
NATIONAL
REHABILITATION
HOSPITAL

THERAPY SERVICES

FORM 200/210-002   8/85

**DAILY
LIVING SKILLS**

FUNCTIONAL PERFORMANCE

EVALUATION

FASTENING DEVICES	Date	10-31		
	Initials	cm		
lace shoes				
fastening shows				
buttons—large/small	c̄ difficulty	3		
zippers—side, front, back				
snaps				
hooks				
suspenders				

comments: Pt demonstrated low frustration tolerance during fine coord activities

ORTHOTICS/PROSTHETICS	Date	10/31		
	Initials	cm		
splints		NA		
brace		NA		
armrest		6		
seat cushion		6		

comments:

COMMUNICATION	Date	10/30		
	Initials	cm		
write name		6		
handle telephone (hold call, hold book, turn pages)		6		
typewriter		NT		
tape recorder		NT		

comments:

MISCELLANEOUS	Date	11/1		
	Initials	cm		
light and hold cigarette		NA		
wind watch and set		NT		
handle money		NT		
pick up object from floor		5		
reach and remove object from tabletop		3		
operate faucets		NT		
operate doors and pass through				
operate elevator				
light switches				
open and close drawer				
use scissors				
electrical outlets				
bed controls				

comments:

BALANCE	Date	11/2		
	Initials	cms		
sitting—unsupported		*		
supported				
standing—unsupported				
supported				

comments: * see obj. data sheet

BED MOBILITY	Date	10/30		
	Initials	cms		
roll to left	SBA	1/5		
roll to right		1		
supine to prone		NT		
prone to supine		NT		
sit to supine	to (L) /(R)	5/LT		
supine to sit	(L) /(R)	5/AT		
bridging		5		

comments: bridging requires min Ⓐ for Ⓡ LE placement; sit → supine c̄ min Ⓐ → mod Ⓐ & v. cues for technique

TRANSFERS	Date	10/31		
	Initials	RV		
bed to chair	SBA c̄ min/mod	5		
chair to bed		5		
chair to toilet	Min/Mod	5		
toilet to chair	Min/Mod	5		
bathtub – shower chair	Min/Mod	5		
to floor		NT		
from floor		NT		

comments: Pt attempted ac̄s tub bench transfer Mod Ⓐ. Requires demonstration cues to complete. Demonstrates impulsivity cm

WHEELCHAIR MOBILITY	Date	10/31		
	Initials	RV		
straight-aways		4		
corners		4		
doors		NT		
inclines				
uneven terrain				
elevators				

comments:

AMBULATION	Date	11/2		
	Initials	cms		
level surfaces		*		
stairs				
inclines				
uneven terrain				
curbs				

comments (gait deviation, device, etc.): * see obj. data sheet

SUMMARY STATEMENT_____

_____

_____

_____

_____

THERAPIST(S):

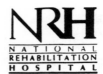

**THERAPY SERVICES
EVALUATION SUMMARY**

PROBLEM	GOAL(S)	TREATMENT PLAN
#1 Self Care	S: Complete TFT as per Dr's orders	Eval. swallowing + self-feeding skills & provide
Ⓐ Feeding	L: To be determined	tx as indicated c̄ possib. referral to SSG,
Ⓑ Dressing	S: Pt will don pullover shirt c̄ Mod Ⓐ + cues	
	L: Pt will complete dressing from wc c̄ Min Ⓐ + min cues overall.	DLS training 2-3x/wk c̄ equipment as indicated
Ⓒ Groom/Hygiene	S: Pt will demonstrate proper use of comb c̄ Min cues + setup	
	L: Completion of bathing + grooming tasks c̄ Min Ⓐ + cues c̄ equipment as needed.	
#2 Functional Mobility	S: Pt will move supine → sit in bed c̄ Mod Ⓐ	
Ⓐ Bed	L: Bed mob. c̄ Min cues	
Ⓑ WC	S: Pt will apply brakes for transfers c̄ reminders	wc mob during functional activities
	L: wc mob c̄ Ⓢ to complete DLS + move about the home	
Ⓒ transfers	S: Pt will complete transfer to/from toilet c̄ Min Ⓐ + cues.	
#3 Work/Leisure	S: Investigate premorbid interests	
	L: Resume activity in premorbid work/leisure tasks c̄ Ⓢ + cues.	
#4 Sensory Motor	S: Pt to participate in PROM exercises	
Ⓐ AROM/PROM	L: Pt to complete AROM exercises c̄ Ⓢ + cues.	

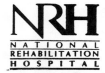

THERAPY SERVICES
EVALUATION SUMMARY

PROBLEM	GOAL(S)	TREATMENT PLAN
Ⓑ Tone	S: Evaluate need for splint to ↓ tone in hand. L: Pt to assist in maintaining tone-inhibiting positioning of Ⓡ UE.	Splint eval + fabrication as indicated Train pt in tone-inhibition technique c̄ equipment
Ⓒ Coordination	S: Pt to participate in Ⓛ UE coord activities & functional tasks L: Use of Ⓛ hand as dominant extremity for functional tasks	fine Coord + functional tasks
Ⓓ Sensory awareness - Ⓡ neglect	S: Pt to attend to Ⓡ side of tray during meals c̄ Min cueing L: Pt to attend to Ⓡ UE/Ⓡ LE, Ⓡ environment c̄ occasional cues.	SSG,
#5 Equipment	S: Equipment eval to be initiated L: DME & small equipment recommendations + train pt in use.	Equipment eval + recs
#7 Cognition	S: Continue eval using functional tasks L: Adequate cognition to complete daily tasks c̄ Min/Mod cueing overall.	Functional Activities Co Tx c̄ SLP
#9 Psychosocial	S/L: Provide support throughout Rehab process. S: Provide tasks to insure small success & thereby ↓ pt frustration level L: Pt will tolerate therapy c̄ Minimal frustration	

THERAPIST(S): _____ 11/3/89
Date

_____ _____ _____
Name Service Date

NRH
N A T I O N A L
R E H A B I L I T A T I O N
H O S P I T A L

THERAPY SERVICES

PROGRESS NOTE
Occupational Therapy ☑

Physical Therapy ☐

Treatment Period: From _11/3/89_ To _11/9/89_

REASON FOR REFERRAL
Primary Medical Diagnosis: _①CVA ®hemiparesis, global aphasia_
Therapy/Treatment Diagnosis: _®hemiparesis, cognitive +_
perceptual deficits

S: _Pt is easily frustrated when completing tasks._

O: For summary of goal accomplishment and status see reverse.

A: Summary statement of functional status including underlying factors and significant issues that impact treatment or attainment of goals: _Pt making small gains in DLS tasks,_
however cognitive/perceptual deficits and inability
to follow verbal commands has limited progress.
It is felt that he will continue to progress
in continued tx. Further it is also necessary
to complete positioning adaptations +
splint to maintain tone inhibiting postures.
Family conference scheduled for 11/14/89

Long term goals met or revised. ☐ No Revisions
New LTGs stated upon completion of
therapeutic feeding program eval
#1A Proper use of utensils, attention to ®
side of tray + maintain normal pace of
eating c̄ occasional cues

Goals reviewed with and agreed upon by patient and/or caregiver
Y ✓ N___

Plan: _Continue toward LTG's as stated in_
eval summary. Begin family training in
equipment needs at time of family
conference.

For summary of goal accomplishment, see reverse side.

Therapist: _____ Date _11/9/89_

Occupational/Physical Therapy Progress Note

Objective tests/measurements (accompaning forms) as well as

Problem #/Title Last Short Term Goal	Goal Met Y/N	Current Status/Comments/Why Goal Not Met	New Short Term Goal
#1A Feeding - Complete TFT	yes	TFT completed - pt results in eval section	Pt will attend to Ⓛ pole of tray č min cues during meals
#1B Dressing - Don pull-over shirt č Mod Ⓐ + cues	yes		
#1C Grooming - Demonstrate proper use of comb č min cues + set up	no	Pt requires Mod cues + setup for proper use of comb č apraxia	Pt will demonstrate proper use of comb č Min cues + setup
#2B Pt will apply yc brakes č reminders for transfers	no	(partially met) Pt requires cues due to locate + apply brake requires verbal + contact guard / min Ⓐ	Pt will apply brakes č reminders before transfers
#2A Bed Mob - Pt will move Ⓐ supine → sit č mod Ⓐ	yes		
#3A Word (review) - not addressed this week			
#4A Sensory Motor - Pt to participate in PROM exercises	yes	Pt able to self range shoulders č demonstration + cues	
#4B Tone - Evaluate need for splint to ↓ tone in hand	yes	Currently fabricating resting hand splint to maintain tone inhibiting position	Pt will tolerate resting hand splint for 4 hour periods daily.
#4C Coordination - Participation in ① OE coordination activities	yes	Pt demonstrate ↑ use of Ⓛ hand during functional tasks (dressing)	
#4D Sensory Awareness - Pt to attend to Ⓛ side of tray during meals č Min cues	no	requires min/mod cues 2° @ field cut	Pt will attend to Ⓛ UE/LE č mod cues during dressing

NRH
NATIONAL
REHABILITATION
HOSPITAL

THERAPY SERVICES

PROGRESS NOTE
Occupational Therapy [✓]

Physical Therapy [ ]

Treatment Period: From 11/9/89   To 11/16/89
REASON FOR REFERRAL
Primary Medical Diagnosis: ⓁCVA c̄ Ⓡ hemiparisis, globalaphasia
Therapy/Treatment Diagnosis: Ⓡ hemiparesis, severe cognitive
& perceptual deficits.

S: _____

O: For summary of goal accomplishment and status see reverse.

A: Summary statement of functional status including underlying
factors and significant issues that impact treatment or attainment
of goals: _Improvement noted in attention to Ⓡ extremete
which had improved patients skill in dressing and
bathing tasks. Pts frustration level during
treatment sessions has ↓'d, allowing him greater
participation in treatment with improved ability
to follow commands. Further treatment is warranted
to order equipment and complete family training
and ↑ Ⓡ UE DLS and complete home evaluation.
family conference held 11/14 and wife & son
signature. They are scheduled to participate in
treatment 11/20/89. Home eval scheduled 11/21/89_

Long term goals met or revised.   [ ] No Revisions

_____
_____
_____
_____
_____
_____
_____

Goals reviewed with and agreed upon by patient and/or caregiver
Y ✗ N ___ _____

Plan: _Continue toward LTG's as stated in
eval summary. Complete home eval. Begin
family training._

For summary of goal accomplishment, see reverse side.

Therapist: _____ Date 11/16/89

Occupational/Physical Therapy Progress Note

Problem #/Title / Last Short Term Goal	Goal Met Y/N	Objective tests/measurements (accompaning forms) as well as / Current Status/Comments/Why Goal Not Met	New Short Term Goal
# 1A. Pt will attend to (R) side of tray c̄ min cues during meals	Yes	Pt requires min/mod cues. It is felt that pt will attain this goal c̄ time	Attend to (R) side of tray c̄ min cues during meals
1B Dressing - no STG stated		Require mod (A) + cues to don clothing	
1C Grooming/Hygiene - Proper use of comb c̄ min cues + setup	No	Partially attained - required min/mod cues + setup	Pt will insert (R) UE through sleeve c̄ Min (A) + cues. Proper use of comb c̄ min cue + set up
2A Bed Mobility no STG		Require CG/Min (A) for supine → sit during DCS routine	Supine → sit c̄ CG/(S) for DCS completion
2B WC Mobility - Pt will apply WC brakes c̄ reminders before transfer	No	Partially attained - requires cues to locate brake	Apply WC brakes c̄ reminders
2C Transfers - no STG		Overall requires Min (A) for bed, tub + toilet transfers c̄ equipment	WC ↔ tub bench transfer c̄ CG/Min (A) + cue
4a Sensory Motor - no STG		Able to perform ROM shoulder c̄ mod cues + (S)	↑ shoulder ROM c̄ min cues to attend to (R) side
4b Bone Pt will tolerate resting hand splint for ? periods	yes	Resting hand splint is effective ē (R) hand - Splint completed + wearing schedule provided to nursing	Pt will tolerate to (R) side. Pt will tolerate splint nightly

NRH

N A T I O N A L
REHABILITATION
H O S P I T A L

THERAPY SERVICES

PROGRESS NOTE
Occupational Therapy ☑

Physical Therapy ☐

Treatment Period: From _11/16/89_ To _11/22/89_

REASON FOR REFERRAL
Primary Medical Diagnosis: _①CVA ® hemiparises, globalaphasia_
Therapy/Treatment Diagnosis: _® weakness severe cognitive_
+ perceptual deficits

S: _Pt appears less agitated during treatment_
sessions

O: For summary of goal accomplishment and status see reverse.

A: Summary statement of functional status including underlying
factors and significant issues that impact treatment or attainment
of goals: _Pt making progress in ® side awareness_
+ DS. Wife has participated in DCS sessions
and in equipment ordering. Further training
is recommended to increase comfort level
c patient. Apraxia + perceptual deficits are
limiting progress to a slow pace. Home eval
completed 11/21/89 - see report in evaluation
sections of chart.

Long term goals met or revised.   ☒ No Revisions

Goals reviewed with and agreed upon by patient and/or caregiver
Y___ N___ _____

Plan: _Complete DME prescriptions._

For summary of goal accomplishment, see reverse side.

Therapist: _____ Date _____

Occupational/Physical Therapy Progress Note

Problem #/Title / Last Short Term Goal	Goal Met Y/N	Objective tests/measurements (accompanying forms) as well as / Current Status/Comments/Why Goal Not Met	New Short Term Goal
1A Feeding Pt will attend to ® side ½ tray ½ min cues	No	Pt requires min/mod cues	mo new goal
1B Dressing Pt will insert ®UE through sleeve ½ min ⒜+ cues	yes		
1C Grooming/Hygiene Pt will use ½ comb ½ min cues + pitey	No	Unable to attain 2° apraxia STG revised	Pt will brush teeth ½ mod ⒜ + cues
2A Bal Mob Supine → Sit ½ CG + cues	yes	Pt requires CG + occasional CG to move ½ supine → sit w/out cues	Pt will move supine → sit ½ ⓢ for D/C completion
2B W/C Mob - Pt will apply w/c brake ½ reminders	No	Partially attained Pt applies brake ½ reminders + cues to locate	Pt will apply w/c brake ½ reminder
2C Transfer - w/c → tub bench ½ CG + min ⒜	yes	Pts wife able to perform/assist ½ transfer	Transfer w/c → toilet CG/ⓢ using program
4A Sensory Motor - Retrograde massage to ®hand	yes	Pt ind effective in edema reduction + tone inhibition Pt tolerate	Pt will perform ®UE in Out/Bed activities
4B Tone Pt will tolerate splint nightly	yes	Splint for 8 hours at night	Pt will weight bearing activities in pitting
4D Sensory Awareness Pt attend to ® side ½ min cues in dressing	yes		Pt will insert ®UE through sleeve ½ min ⒜ + cues

NRH
NATIONAL
REHABILITATION
HOSPITAL

THERAPY SERVICES

PROGRESS NOTE
Occupational Therapy ☒

Physical Therapy ☐

Treatment Period: From ___11/22/89___ To ___11/29/89___

REASON FOR REFERRAL
Primary Medical Diagnosis: _①CVA ® hemiparesis_
Therapy/Treatment Diagnosis: _① side weakness, global_
aphasia, cognitive/perceptual deficits

S: _∅_

O: For summary of goal accomplishment and status see reverse.

A: Summary statement of functional status including underlying
factors and significant issues that impact treatment or attainment
of goals: _Pt continues to make slow steady_
progress in PCS + awareness of ① side during
functional tasks. ↓ impulsivity, + ↑ frustration
tolerance. Further training is necessary to
↑ ① c̄ PCS, further family training + complete
equipment training.

Long term goals met or revised. ☐ No Revisions

#2A Bed Mobility c̄ min cues attained

Goals reviewed with and agreed upon by patient and/or caregiver
Y _✓_ N___ _____

Plan: _____
Work on LTG's as stated in eval
summary.

For summary of goal accomplishment, see reverse side.

Therapist:_____ Date_____

Occupational/Physical Therapy Progress Note

Objective tests/measurements (accompaning forms) as well as

Problem #/Title / Last Short Term Goal	Goal Met Y/N	Current Status/Comments/Why Goal Not Met	New Short Term Goal
#1A+7 Feeding/Cognition / Attend to (L) side of tray	yes	Req. min (A) + cue to don / shirt over (R)UE	Program ind. to visual + occasional cues
1B Dressing/(R)upper/lower / front (R)UE through sleeve	yes	Requires pt up to / dressing task	Pt will stand + raise / pants c (R)UE + cues
1C Grooming Brush teeth	yes	min/mod (A) → cues	
2A Bed Mob.- supine→pt / c supervision	yes	STG attained	
2B W/C Mob.- apply / brakes c reminders	yes		Pt will propel w/c to / obtain DC's items c / verbal cues
2C transfers w/c ↔ toilet / c (R)G using UE frame	yes		
3 Wash/dress (R)w STG		Pt refuses to participate will / attempt again	
4A ROM - Partion (R)UE in / wb activities in sitting	MO	Now tolerating weight / bearing c ↑ ability to / follow through	Continue c stated / STG
4D Sensory Awareness / (R)UE through sleeve c / min (A) + cues	yes		
5 Equipment - Complete / DME prescription	yes		

Follow-Up Questions for Chapter 13

Now that you have reviewed Cases A and B, and performed the review of Case C with the CRF, did you notice the following:

1. that written physician orders were not present in all three cases?
2. that Case C contained a format that made tracking the goals and the patient's performance easy to follow?
3. that in Cases A and C, minimal note-writing time was required from the therapist, but the treatment elements were adequately documented?
4. that in Cases B and C, the long-term and short-term goals were oriented to patient activity performance?
5. that in Cases B and C, it appears that the patient and/or caregiver were interviewed by the therapist as to the requested goals for occupational therapy?
6. that in all three cases, the documentation was sufficiently adequate in its content for the claim to be paid?

With these considerations in mind, a good exercise would be to take samples of your own patient documentation and use the CRF to perform a review.

14. Legal Issues in Documentation: Fraud, Abuse, and Confidentiality

Thomas Steich

As we document the case of each patient or client, the immediate reasons for our notes, such as good communication, are obvious. This author discusses how important clear documentation can be years later. He also discusses the important federal and state laws affecting documentation and related practices.

Thomas Steich is general counsel for the American Occupational Therapy Association.

The act of creating a document may result in unintended consequences. The other chapters of this book describe many positive reasons for documentation. This chapter will discuss the "risky" side of documentation, which is the creation of a "smoking gun" of evidence that may prove intentional or unintentional violations of law.

The documentation generated by occupational therapy personnel is subject to many laws and regulations once created. This chapter will discuss two of the most important laws, those prohibiting fraud and abuse and those protecting the patient's right of privacy, because these laws impose certain duties on the creator and custodian of the documents. Occupational therapy personnel must be aware of these duties.

General Record Keeping Considerations

Good record keeping can help to avoid or win medical malpractice lawsuits. Most lawsuits are filed many years after the medical care was provided. Juries find it difficult to believe that care was rendered if it is not documented.

One must prepare complete records. Complete records help jog your memory so that you can remember one particular patient from all of your patients if you should be asked to give testimony.

Requirements

When recording information, always tell the truth and complete the record at the time of treatment or as soon as possible thereafter. The more time that elapses between treatment and recording, the greater the possibility of error. Time and date all entries. Use specific rather than general terms. Use quotations to document unusual or bizarre patient behavior. Record broken appointments and patient "no shows" with reasons given by the patient and describe any attempts to reschedule appointments.

Do not do any of the following:

- change a record after the fact without clarifying when the change was made and the nature of the change
- criticize another health care provider in a written record
- make judgmental statements about a patient or patient's family instead of a factual statement. For example, "Patient claims he is from Mars," states a fact while "Patient is crazy" states a judgment.
- assume the patient will not see the medical records.

Use of Medical Record

Medical records are evidence of medical treatment provided to a patient. They are used as evidence in court proceedings, administrative hearings such as Workers Compensation and Social Security hearings, and legislative proceedings. A therapist who performed the services described in the medical record or who has custody of the record may be called to testify in any of these proceedings about the medical record. Therefore it is vital that the records be documented truthfully and accurately.

The Medical Record as a Legal Document

All of the purposes of documentation are important. The first purpose, however, provides the link between occupational therapy practitioners and their environment. It focuses on the legal requirements for documentation. As a legal document, the medical record is the form of communication that health professionals use to communicate with the larger society in which they practice.

There are numerous laws with slight variations and professional standards that govern documentation. Both state and federal laws require health care providers to maintain records on the patients or clients they treat. Some of these laws are Medicare, Medicaid, state laws governing medical records, privacy acts, and licensure laws. All practitioners must know which laws affect their practice in order to meet the requirements of these laws and to document their services effectively. The Medicare law is usually the most stringent, so following its requirements will usually suffice to meet standards set in other guidelines. Each practitioner must be responsible for identifying and meeting the specific requirements in his or her state.

As you have read elsewhere, Medicare requires that treatment result in *practical* improvement within a reasonable period of time. Documentation must describe a *skilled* service. The practitioner must show that the skills of an occupational therapist are required to perform the service.

Effective documentation is essential for third party payment. It itemizes the frequency, duration, and nature of services delivered. Upon request, the practitioner must be ready to demonstrate the specific service delivered. Without proper medical records to verify payment for services, a payer can deny reimbursement and even seek to recover past payments. If a payer suspects fraud or abuse in billing for services, and medical records are found to be inaccurate, fictitious, or "doctored" to generate improper payments, the providers are subject to prosecution and possible criminal penalties. The federal government has enforced the Medicare "Fraud and Abuse" law against health care providers to recover Medicare payments that were illegally paid to providers.

Similar liabilities are found in Medicaid and private health insurance contracts. The best defense against improper billing actions by a payer is to maintain accurate and complete documentation of all services delivered. If practitioners follow the guidelines and terminology specified by the payer in the medical record, it is unlikely that questions will arise or that services will not be covered.

You should be careful *not* to cosign another person's notes for reimbursement unless you supervised that person and they are providing occupational therapy services. A therapist should use only qualified persons to provide treatment. The use of occupational therapy aides varies from state to state; therefore, check with your third party payers and your state regulatory laws.

Medicare and Medicaid Fraud and Abuse

For those readers in private practice the following section is of particular importance. Since Congress enacted the Medicare and Medicaid Programs in 1965, it has enacted legislation in 1972, 1977, and 1987 to facilitate the discovery and prevention of fraud and abuse in these programs. The 1977 legislation added Section 1128B(b) of the Social Security Act to provide criminal penalties for various kickbacks, bribes, or rebate practices involving Medicare and Medicaid. These provisions prohibit payments that are in return for or intended to induce the referral of Medicare or Medicaid business.

In other words, individuals or entities that knowingly and willfully offer, pay, solicit, or receive remuneration in order to induce business reimbursed under Medicare or Medicaid are guilty of a felony punishable by fines and imprisonment.

This prohibition is extremely broad. The types of remuneration covered specifically include kickbacks, bribes, and rebates made directly or indirectly, overtly or covertly, in cash or in kind. In addition, prohibited conduct includes not only remuneration intended to induce referrals of patients, but also remuneration intended to induce the purchasing, leasing, ordering, or arranging for any good, facility, service, or item paid by Medicare or Medicaid health care programs.

The leading case regarding this law illustrates its broad prohibition. In *United States v. Greber* (1985), the Federal Third Circuit Court of Appeals was asked to examine the nature of payments between a medical diagnostic company, providing Holter monitor services, and physicians. The company billed Medicare for the monitoring service it performed and forwarded 40% of those payments (up to $65 per patient) to the referring physician.

The defendant claimed that these payments were merely interpretation fees paid to the referring physicians for their initial consultation and for explaining the test results to the patients. The court, however, refused to examine whether there might have been a legitimate purpose behind the payments and ruled that if one purpose of the payment is to induce future referrals, the medicare statute has been violated (*United States v. Greber*, 1985).

Because the Fraud and Abuse law is so broad in its prohibition, many health care providers are concerned that innocuous or even beneficial commercial arrangements are technically covered by the law and subject to criminal prosecution.

1987 Amendments

Public Law 100-93, the Medicare and Medicaid Patient and Program Protection Act of 1987, added two new provisions addressing the anti-kickback statute. Section 2 gives authority to the Office of Inspector General (OIG) to exclude a person or entity from participation in the Medicare and Medicaid health care programs if they engaged in a prohibited remuneration scheme. This new civil remedy is intended to provide an alternative to criminal prosecution that will be more effective in regulating abusive business practices than criminal prosecution.

In addition, section 14 of the law attempts to address the concerns of providers by requiring the promulgation of "safe harbor" regulations specifying those payment practices that will not be subject to criminal prosecution under the Act and that will not provide a basis for exclusion from the Medicare and Medicaid programs.

In January 1989, the U.S. Department of Health and Human Services (HHS) issued proposed "safe harbor" regulations specifying which payment practices are immune from the civil, criminal, and other sanctions of the Federal Medicare and Medicaid anti-kickback statute in January 1989 (42 CFR, part 1001, Subpart E). These regulations became effective July 29, 1991. The "safe harbors" cover the following payment practices:

- investment interests
- space rental
- equipment rental
- personal services and management contracts
- sale of practice
- referral services
- warranties
- discounts
- employees
- group purchasing organizations.

It may be impossible to provide services without seeking the legal advice of an attorney concerning compliance with this anti-kickback law. There is uncertainty about whether these "safe harbor" regulations will reduce the risk to providers.

The intent of the Medicare Prospective Payment system enacted in 1984 was to encourage hospital cost-effectiveness and competitive strategies, many of which have a partial goal of increasing referral patterns. However, the broad language of the Medicare fraud statutes and of the previously mentioned court case *United States v. Greber* (1985) conflict with the competitive incentives by prohibiting payments intended to induce the referral of Medicare or Medicaid business. Physician recruitment programs, physician incentive plans, hospital-physician joint ventures, shared service agreements, and hospital waivers of coinsurance have all been challenged as illegal inducements. Therapists should assume their commercial arrangements with physicians and hospitals may be challenged by the government.

Occupational therapy personnel must become familiar with these safe harbor regulations to reduce their risk. Other steps they can take are to structure their Medicare/Medicaid business within guidelines obtained from past HHS advisory opinions, intermediary letters, and other informal sources. For a more detailed explanation of the issues confronting private practitioners and Medicare/Medicaid Fraud & Abuse Law, see chapter 7 of AOTA's *Private Practice Manual* (Hertfelder & Crispen, 1990, chap. 7).

Patient Confidentiality Laws

A majority of states have enacted Medical Records Confidentiality Statutes to protect confidential information involving personal medical records, hospital records, or research records from disclosure. There is some conflict between these laws and the Medicare/Medicaid Anti-Kickback laws.

The Medicare and Medicaid programs have been plagued by health care providers' fraudulent and abusive practices since their enactment in 1965. To help states discover and prevent Medicare and Medicaid fraud, Congress has enacted laws permitting access to patients' medical records in fraud investigations. The majority of states have enacted physician-patient and psychotherapist-patient privilege statutes to protect confidential information from disclosure. The state's need for patient information conflicts with the patient's right of privacy. After balancing the state interest in eliminating fraud against the patient's privacy interest, the courts have often allowed disclosure of patient medical records. Although some courts have attempted to limit the extent of the information disclosed, few have provided specific standards to protect patient records from unwarranted disclosure of confidential information.

State patient confidentiality laws are divided into those governing research records and those governing personal medical records.

Confidential Research Records

A "confidential research record" is any record, report, statement, note, or other information that is assembled or obtained for research or study and names or otherwise identifies any person. Its custody and use are generally restricted. The confidential record may only be used for the research and study for which it was assembled or obtained. The records can only be disclosed to persons engaged in the research or study project.

The only exception allowing for disclosure to others is an aggregate summary that does not disclose the identity of any person who is the subject of the confidential record. Confidential Research Record laws usually apply to public health departments and drug abuse agencies and their agents.

Personal Medical Records

Occupational therapy personnel in their practices are more likely to come into contact with laws regulating the disclosure of personal medical records because occupational therapy personnel are more involved with patient care than with research, and these laws apply to any provider of medical care, whether the provider is an individual or an organization.

What is a medical record will depend on the legal definitions found in your state law. At a minimum, the definition covers every record of medical care that a health care provider or facility maintains on an individual. This includes any document that clearly identifies a patient by name, number, age, and sex; shows clearly the services provided; when, where, and by whom; the diagnosis and prognosis; and the treatment, therapy, and health status of the patient.

These laws provide for authorized disclosures under limited circumstances, prohibit disclosures unless authorized by the individual on whom the record is kept, distinguish between records kept by individuals and records kept by facilities, and establish timelines and procedures for the destruction of the medical records.

The Maryland law (Health General Article, Title 4, Subtitle 3) provides a good example of a state Medical Records Confidentiality law. Under the Maryland law, the medical records of an adult patient may not be destroyed for 5 years after the record is made. The records of a minor patient may not be destroyed for 5 years after the record is made or until the patient attains the age of 21, whichever is later, unless the parent or guardian is notified.

It should be noted that with respect to hospital records the standard of the Joint Commission on Accreditation of Healthcare Organizations (JCAHO) is exceptionally vague and provides little guidance on when to destroy. Consequently, the policy of most hospitals is to retain patient records forever.

The record cannot be disclosed without the patient's consent except for situations including performing medical services on the patient, medical peer review, pursuant to legal process or lawful request by the government, pursuant to a medical research protocol, pursuant to a malpractice claim, providing information to a third party payer for billing purposes, and for organ donation purposes.

References

Hertfelder, S., & Crispen, C. (Eds.). (1990). *Private practice: Strategies for success.* Rockville, MD: American Occupational Therapy Association.

United States v. Greber, 760 F.2d 68 (3d Cir.), cert. denied, 474 U.S. 988, 106 S. Ct. 396 (1985).

15. Ethical Issues in Documentation

Sharon Reitz, MS, OTR

This chapter concludes the book with a discussion of the important relationship of documentation to ethical issues. The American Occupational Therapy Association has made a serious effort through its Code of Ethics *and other documents discussed in this chapter to give ethical issues the prominence they deserve.*

Sharon Reitz is an assistant professor in the occupational therapy department, Towson State University, Towson, MD.

The preceding chapter discussed the legal aspects of documentation. That discussion was based on current laws and statutes that have developed over time from ethical principles, most commonly from principles of justice. The American Occupational Therapy Association's (AOTA's) *Occupational Therapy Code of Ethics* is based upon these principles as well as others, and it serves to guide both the practice of occupational therapy and the documentation of that practice. This chapter briefly discusses the historical interest of occupational therapy in quality documentation and familiarizes the reader with various ethical principles promoted by AOTA, AOTA's Standards and Ethics Commission (SEC), and the American Occupational Therapy Certification Board (AOTCB). Most importantly, the chapter outlines a process for resolving ethical dilemmas and concludes with a discussion of actual documentation issues in a case study format.

The importance of gaining both knowledge and skill in documentation has long been appreciated by the profession of occupational therapy. As early as 1948, *The American Journal of Occupational Therapy (AJOT)* published an article on documentation (Booth,1948). Through the years, articles on the legal and ethical aspects of documentation (Gleave, 1960) as well on specific documentation skills (Carr, 1969; Overs, 1964) have appeared in *AJOT*. These articles can be relevant and applicable to current practice. Overs provided a succinct review of documenting work evaluations, a popular and growing segment of occupational therapy practice in the 1990s.

The AOTA's *Code of Ethics* requires that members of the association examine the quality of both their practice and the documentation that reflects that practice. In recent years, financial constraints and the resulting increased scrutiny by fiscal intermediaries have further stimulated interest in documentation issues and quality assurance processes.

This is demonstrated by the increasing number of items published on documentation. A computerized search using OT SOURCE (AOTA, 1989) listed 11 entries under the heading "documentation" for 1988, half of them focusing on reimbursement issues. Prior to 1988, the annual number of entries ranged from zero to three. The case studies presented in this chapter reflect the current focus on documentation. Prior to reading the case studies, the reader should become familiar with the AOTA's *Code of Ethics* (see Chapter Appendix A) and *Reference Guide* (AOTA, 1991), the SEC's *Enforcement Procedure for Occupational Therapy Code of Ethics* (see Chapter Appendix B), and the AOTCB's *Procedures for Disciplinary Action* (see Chapter Appendix C). The reader should also become familiar with a systematic process for resolving ethical issues. A detailed discussion of ethical theories, principles, and general terms can be found in the May 1988 *AJOT* special issue on ethics, especially in its article on ethical reasoning (Kyler-Hutchison, 1988).

Ethical Reasoning Process

There are different ways to analyze ethical dilemmas. One process will be described and demonstrated in this chapter. Even when individuals use the same process, they may arrive at different conclusions based on their value systems. Therefore, therapists must be conscious of potential conflicts in values, viewpoints, and needs among health care providers (Hansen, 1988). It is important for each therapist to consciously examine the dilemmas that arise and consider a variety of possible courses of action prior to making a decision. Action should not be taken on impulse, which can occur when highly regarded values are threatened. When threatened, people tend to react in an immediate and exaggerated manner (Everly, 1990), which frequently results in responses that may seem irrational to others and may be hard to defend. A more professional response to an ethical dilemma will be formulated if the decision: (a) has been carefully analyzed and executed, (b) is consistent with the therapist's personal value system, (c) is compatible with the laws and regulations to which the therapist is bound, and (d) is executed only after all available options are considered.

The case studies in this chapter use a 5-step process (Aroskar, 1980; Hansen, Kamp, & Reitz, 1988), outlined in Table 15.1. During the process of resolving ethical dilemmas it is important to be open and receptive to contrasting points of view. Competent

Table 15.1 Steps in an ethical reasoning process

---

1. Gather All Additional Pertinent Information

First, identify the "players" or participants in the dilemma. Next, gather information regarding the specific dilemma and review the AOTA's *Code of Ethics*, the *Enforcement Procedure* of AOTA's SEC, and the AOTCB's *Procedures for Disciplinary Action*, as well as the code of ethics and the documentation guidelines of the institution/workplace. Documentation and practice guidelines of fiscal intermediaries should also be reviewed.

2. Identify Conflicting Values and Neutral Territory

Time needs to be taken to identify possible conflicting values between the participants, as well as values that may be compatible if not identical. Locating this neutral territory of shared values may facilitate the resolution of the dilemma.

3. Identify All Possible Alternative Actions

All alternatives should be listed—even those that at the beginning may seem risky or inappropriate. The commitment to the final choice of action might be strengthened by a clear understanding of the reasons for and the consequences of the alternative actions. The therapist may also find this preparation helpful if it becomes necessary to defend the final choice to others.

4. Determine Both Positive and Negative Consequences of Each Action

A realistic appraisal of the costs and benefits of each possible action should be listed so that they can be reviewed at length.

5. Weigh the Actions and Their Consequences to Determine the Best Possible Course of Action

Sufficient time should be taken to carefully weigh the total positive and negative consequences of each action and all possible combinations of actions to select an action that is both "right" and defensible.

Sources: Adapted from Aroskar, 1980; Hansen, Kamp, & Reitz, 1988

therapists should be aware of their value systems and the potential areas of conflict within their particular workplaces. Therapists are also responsible for being familiar with all federal and state laws and regulations that govern their practice.

When a dilemma arises, the occupational therapist should first identify the "players" involved. Next, all necessary information about legal and professional standards should be gathered. The therapist must become familiar with the laws and regulations that pertain to the particular issue and practice area. Copies of the following should be obtained for guidance: AOTA's *Code of Ethics* and *Reference Guide*, the *Enforcement Procedure* of AOTA's SEC, the AOTCB's *Procedures for Disciplinary Action*, as well as any written documents from the state's regulatory board, if appropriate. After all additional pertinent and accessible information has been gathered, the occupational therapist should determine whether any conflicting values between participants can be identified.

If an employer determines that treatment is no longer cost-effective, regardless of the patient's progress as measured and documented by the therapist, the therapist must choose between conflicting values. The therapist may be caught between the value of upholding a duty to the patient, the principle of nonmaleficence (i.e., doing no harm), and the value of upholding a duty to an employer. It is not always possible to identify conflicting values initially. The true nature of a dilemma will become more apparent when the conflicts are identified. Most often, ethical dilemmas are complex, and a variety of values are involved. It may be helpful to identify those areas where conflicting parties share similar values and goals. Locating this neutral territory or middle ground is an important first step. Once it has been identified, a collaborative problem-solving effort that allows mutual respect for differing values is possible.

The next step in the ethical reasoning process consists of listing all possible actions or responses to the dilemma. Skills in problem solving are an asset here. The quality of the final resolution of the dilemma is dependent upon the variety and comprehensiveness of alternative actions that can be developed.

Next, the consequences—both positive and negative—of each possible action should be determined. Finally, all of the options and their consequences should be weighed and balanced. The action that best coincides with the therapist's value system should be selected as the optimal course of action. By following this or a similar ethical reasoning process, a thoughtful solution can be articulated and defended. This process will be applied in the following two case analyses. The analyses of these cases are not exhaustive but rather are illustrative examples used for educational purposes.

Application of Ethical Reasoning Process

An expert in the field provided the information about the most frequently reported dilemmas faced by practicing occupational therapists upon which these fictitious cases are based (C. Crispen, personal communication, January 29 & 31, 1990). These case studies were discussed informally with other experts in the field, and their feedback was used in the development of the lists of possible alternative actions.

Case Study One

The director of occupational therapy, a registered occupational therapist, announced at a staff meeting that staff occupational therapists will be cosigning notes for the art and dance therapists in the future. When asked why, she said that this practice would ensure that these services would be reimbursed as occupational therapy by third party payers and that the hospital needed to ensure that adequate funds were provided by reimbursement mechanisms in order to provide quality services. One therapist was concerned about both the legal and ethical implications of this new policy. What should this therapist do?

First, the therapist should gather additional, pertinent facts and information from all parties involved, as well as the appropriate documents. The therapist can initiate this process by reviewing AOTA's *Code of Ethics* and *Reference Guide*. In addition, the therapist should review the documentation guidelines of the third party payers involved. It may also be helpful to investigate the ethical code and standards of practice of the art and dance therapists. When discussing ethics there are only opposing views, not a "right" view and a "wrong" view. However, when fraud is present (i.e., billing a non–occupational therapy service as occupational therapy), the issue becomes a legal one. Fraudulent billing is unlawful and therefore unethical according to the AOTA's *Code of Ethics* and the AOTCB's *Procedures for Disciplinary Action*. However, the manner in which both the dilemma and the original problem are resolved (i.e., reimbursement for non–occupational therapy services) depends on ethical reasoning. Possible alternative actions may vary depending on personal and institutional values and viewpoints.

The next step in the ethical reasoning process is to construct a table similar to Table 15.2, which displays steps 3 and 4 in the ethical reasoning process for the case study. The major tools needed for the final analysis of the ethical dilemma are displayed in this table. Time should then be spent studying the options outlined in the table, weighing the value of each alternative action and determining which action or combination of actions would be most consistent with the therapist's personal value system and the AOTA's *Code of Ethics*. Gathering the appropriate information and educating people about the ramifications of their behavior or proposed behavior (Action #3) are often sufficient to resolve ethical dilemmas. The other alternative actions listed in the tables should be considered only as last resorts.

A general rule in resolving ethical dilemmas is that attempts to resolve the dilemma should begin at the level closest to the participants. Attempts should be made to resolve this particular dilemma with the director before escalating the situation by reporting the director to the appropriate regulatory board (e.g., state regulatory board, AOTA's SEC, or AOTCB). The AOTA has jurisdiction

Table 15.2 Case study one: Analysis of alternative actions

Action	**Consequences**
1. Follow director's proposal without asking any questions or seeking additional information.	*Positive*: Less risky in the short term. *Negative*: Risk of engaging in illegal and unethical conduct; in opposition to AOTA's *Code of Ethics*—Principles 3A, 3B, 3D, & 6; against personal values.
2. Report director immediately to reimbursement agencies.	*Positive*: Fraudulent billing will be stopped/not initiated. *Negative*: In opposition to AOTA's *Code of Ethics*—Principle 3B; disruptive to relationship with supervisor.
3. Request to meet with the director after reviewing the following additional information: Third Party Payment Guidelines AOTA's *Code of Ethics* AOTCB's *Procedures for Disciplinary Action* Art/Dance Therapy Code of Ethics/Standards of Practice	*Positive*: Supported by AOTA's *Code of Ethics*—Principles 3B, 3D, 4B, & 6; increases personal knowledge of ethics, codes of ethics, and regulations and enhances ability to educate supervisor. *Negative:* May be risky if director is not in agreement; meeting may become confrontational.
4. If the director is prepared to rescind the policy, provide support as needed and develop possible alternative strategies, for example: • Investigate if OTRs periodically evaluate patients' progress, can this service be legally billed? (This may be an additional source for reimbursed services.) • Investigate whether co-led groups (i.e., OTR and art/dance therapists) can be billed for? • Conduct quality assurance studies to determine the effectiveness of art/dance therapy in this setting by collecting data as to whether patients who receive art and dance therapy and OT meet treatment goals and are discharged quicker than those just receiving OT. • Contact the professional associations for art/dance therapy to determine if the hospital can assist in their efforts to become a reimbursable service. • If any art or dance therapists express an interest in graduate school, introduce them to OT schools with degrees for non-OTs.	*Positive*: Supported by AOTA's *Code of Ethics*—Principles 3B, 3D, 4B, & 6; supportive of director. *Negative*: May be risky in terms of job security.
5. If director does not take action, discuss issue with hospital administrator.	*Positive:* Supported by AOTA's *Code of Ethics*—Principles 3B, 5, & 6; increases understanding of codes.

Continued on opposite page

Table 15.2 (continued)

	Negative: Risk to job security; disloyalty to director.
6. Inform the director that you are prepared to make a report to the appropriate regulatory board (i.e., state regulatory board, AOTA's SEC commission, or AOTCB). Follow through with report if necessary.	*Positive*: Supported by AOTA's *Code of Ethics*—Principles 3B, 3D, 4B, 5, & 6. *Negative*: Risk to job security; disloyalty to director.
7. If the hospital does not take action, meet again with the administrator and inform him or her that you are prepared to report the hospital to the reimbursement agency's fraud section. If action is still not taken, follow through with report.	*Positive*: Supported by AOTA's *Code of Ethics*—Principles 3B, 3D, 4B, 5, & 6. *Negative*: Risk to job security; disloyalty to director and hospital.
8. If director does not take action, quit without taking any action.	*Positive*: Remove personal risk of legal repercussions. *Negative*: Disloyalty to director and patients; in opposition to AOTA's *Code of Ethics*—Principle 5.

only over its members. If the director is not a member of AOTA, it would not be appropriate to make a report to AOTA's SEC; however, since she is a registered occupational therapist, it would be appropriate to contact the AOTCB. The benefits of resolving dilemmas prior to reporting to an external authority include: (a) increasing the probability that the dilemma may be resolved quickly; (b) providing an approach compatible with Principle 3B of the AOTA's *Code of Ethics*, which states that therapists are responsible for informing "colleagues about those laws and policies that apply to the profession" (AOTA, 1988, p. 795); (c) educating the staff and administration concerning the effects of ethical dilemmas on practice; and (d) enhancing the therapist's credibility (i.e., the fact that the therapist "went through channels") if the disagreement is escalated.

In one resolution of this case, the therapist, after carefully studying the options, attempts to educate the director regarding the issues of fraud (see Table 15.2—Action #3). In selecting this action, the therapist has weighed the value of upholding duties to: the employer (i.e., director and institution), the profession's code of ethics, and the law. At first it may seem that these values are in conflict; however, all of these values support Action #3. Principle 3B of the AOTA's *Code of Ethics* clearly gives the therapist guidance in selecting this option. It is important that the therapist establish a collaborative rather than a confrontational tone when meeting with the director and/or hospital administration. The common goal of providing quality treatment while maintaining fiscal responsibility should be stressed. It is important during the resolution of any ethical dilemma to find middle ground or a common goal, which can enhance collaboration and the potential for a successful resolution.

The majority of cases can be satisfactorily resolved using this approach. If, however, this strategy proves unsuccessful, the therapist needs to carefully weigh the other possible courses of action presented in Table 15.2. These alternative actions (Actions # 5–8) should be used only as a last resort after repeated unsuccessful attempts to educate the director and the hospital administration. Their greater potential consequences include the possibility of: (a) limiting treatments and services or jeopardizing the institution's accreditation and reimbursement sources because of illegal practices and (b) losing a job or engaging in fraudulent billing and losing one's credentials to practice occupational therapy

If the hospital adopts the proposed policy—resulting in the director being engaged in fraud—the therapist is bound by the AOTA's *Code of Ethics* to report the director's behavior to an appropriate regulatory body (i.e., AOTCB, AOTA's SEC, or state regulatory board). AOTA and AOTCB have no jurisdiction over the hospital administrator or the hospital as a whole. The AOTA's *Code of Ethics* supports the therapist in reporting the hospital administration to the appropriate authorities (i.e., the fraud section of the fiscal intermediaries). Prior to reporting either party, the therapist should inform both the director and the hospital administrator of this plan and provide them with the opportunity to reconsider their decisions.

This is one of many possible resolutions of this hypothetical dilemma. Occupational therapists, who are skilled in problem solving, communication, and task analysis, can be extremely adept at resolving both dilemmas and management crises in an ethical and cost-effective manner. The proposed strategies that could be substituted for the process of having the registered occupational therapists cosign the notes (Action #3) are an example of this problem-solving approach.

Case Study Two   The chief of an occupational therapy department, in which two of six therapists are on maternity leave, was informed by one of the remaining therapists that he and his spouse would be moving out of state in 1 month. The chief approached the hospital administrator to request more funding for recruitment. The administrator suggested that more creative approaches be developed to solve the temporary staffing shortage. Specifically, the administrator suggested that the chief train three of the hospital's nursing aides to provide occupational therapy services until the two therapists return from maternity leave. Once the therapists returned, the chief could then select the aide with the best performance record as a permanent occupational therapy technician. "Quite a satisfactory arrangement, don't you agree?" the administrator asked. How should the chief of occupational therapy respond?

Now that the reader is familiar with the format and process of ethical reasoning that is being used, the rest of the case will be presented in a more concise form. Table 15.3 lists the alternative actions and consequences for the second case.

It is important for the chief to refrain from making premature judgments (e.g., "All the administrator ever thinks about is

Table 15.3 Case study two: Analysis of alternative actions

Action	Consequences
1. Follow administrator's directions without asking any questions or seeking additional information.	*Positive*: Less risky for job security. *Negative*: Risk of engaging in illegal or unethical conduct in opposition to AOTA's *Code of Ethics*—Principles 1H, 3A, 3B, 3D, & 6; against personal values.
2. State that you have concerns about the legality and ethics of this solution. Suggest you meet again after you have reviewed the possible ramifications.	*Positive*: Supported by AOTA's *Code of Ethics*—Principles 3A & 3B. *Negative*: May be risky to job security if administrator is not concerned about legal or ethical issues.
3. Quit after determining that fraud could be involved (i.e., if service provided by non-OT is billed as OT).	*Negative*: In opposition to AOTA's *Code of Ethics*—Principle 3B; administrator's solution may be instituted upon your departure, putting staff and patients at risk.
4a. Investigate alternate strategies to present to administrator, for example: • Investigate use of on-call OTR/temporary OTR. • Suggest that the use of technicians be restricted to maintenance therapy, which cannot be billed as OT; when the patients *are* reevaluated by an OTR, that session can be charged as OT. • Investigate a policy of priority scheduling. • Investigate possibility of decreasing frequency of therapy sessions to ensure that all priority patients are treated, with technicians to provide carry-over activities on the days that patients do not receive therapy.	*Positive*: Displays leadership skills and skills in resolving ethical dilemmas through problem solving. *Negative*: Takes time away from other administrative and clinical duties.
4b. Meet with administrator and present alternative actions (see 4a above) and additional concerns, such as: What is the cost, in terms of both time and money, to train these technicians? What duties will they be competent to perform? How will their competency be determined? How will their activities be documented and charged for? Since additional training will be required, will this be viewed as a promotion? Will the salary of the technicians increase from that of their current job?	*Positive*: Supported by AOTA's *Code of Ethics*—Principles 1H, 3A, 3B, 3C, 3D, & 4B. *Negative*: May be risky to job security if administrator is not concerned about legal or ethical issues; meeting may get confrontational.

Continued on opposite page

Table 15.3 (continued)

Are there opportunities for further career upward mobility? Will this be a cost-effective solution if implemented in a legal fashion?

5. If administrator wants to institute his solution, including fraudulent billing, quit.	*Positive*: Supported by AOTA's *Code of Ethics*—Principles 4B, 5A, & 6. *Negative*: Risk of losing job reference; disloyalty to staff and patients.
6. If administrator wants to institute his solution, including fraudulent billing, meet again and inform administrator that you are prepared to report him to the fraud sections of the appropriate third party payers. Follow through with reports if issue is not resolved.	*Positive*: Supported by AOTA's *Code of Ethics*—Principles 3B, 3D, 4B, 5A, & 6. *Negative*: Risk of losing job.

money!") or allowing initial impressions to cloud the analysis of the dilemma (e.g., "I guess he has checked into the legalities and I'd better go along or I'll be out the door."). The chief should take the time to logically consider the dilemma. Again, the first step would be to gather additional pertinent information listed in Table 15.3—Action #2.

By following an ethical reasoning process, the chief found that the AOTA's *Code of Ethics*, Principle 4B (AOTA, 1988) prohibits fraudulent communication and that billing services provided by individuals who are neither registered occupational therapists nor certified occupational therapy assistants can be considered fraudulent under Medicare guidelines. Additionally, the chief became aware that Medicare and other fiscal intermediaries are actively searching for this type of fraud (C. Crispen, personal communication, January 29 & 31, 1990). It also became clear that both the chief and technicians would be committing fraud if their services were billed as occupational therapy services.

After reviewing the values and goals of the occupational therapy department and the administrator's goals, several creative solutions became apparent, which are listed in Table 15.3—Action #4a. Several questions—aside from the question of billing—also came into focus as the chief examined the issue (see Table 15.3—Action #4b). As has been stated before, in the majority of cases, having clear, predetermined, and well-articulated questions and alternative solutions when meeting with superiors leads to successful and productive outcomes. Only as a last resort should more vigorous actions be required.

In closing this chapter, it should be stressed that competent documentation can be a powerful tool in both communicating a patient's response to therapy and also educating other health care providers and fiscal intermediaries to the value of occupational therapy. Incompetent, unethical, or fraudulent documentation, on the other hand, puts the therapist at risk of facing legal repercussions and diminishes the credibility and potential of the profession as a whole. Documentation must not be viewed as a nuisance, waste of time, luxury, or purely intellectual/academic exercise. It is an integral part of competent clinical practice. Documentation must be pursued with vigor and commitment so that the profession can continue to respond to the potential recipients of occupational therapy services.

References

American Occupational Therapy Association. (1988). Occupational therapy code of ethics. *American Journal of Occupational Therapy, 42,* 795-796.

American Occupational Therapy Association Standards and Ethics Commission. (1988). *Enforcement procedure for occupational therapy code of ethics.* Rockville, MD: Author.

American Occupational Therapy Association. (1989). *Alphamate for OT SOURCE* [Computer program]. Rockville, MD: Author.

American Occupational Therapy Association. (1991). *Reference guide: Occupational therapy code of ethics.* Rockville, MD: Author.

American Occupational Therapy Certification Board. (1991). *Procedures for disciplinary action.* Rockville, MD: Author.

Aroskar, M. (1980). Anatomy of an ethical dilemma: The practice (Part II). *American Journal of Nursing, 80,* 661-663.

Booth, M. (1948). An occupational therapist's guide for progress notes: Which facts and why. *American Journal of Occupational Therapy, 2,* 15-19.

Carr, S. (1969). Documentation of services. *American Journal of Occupational Therapy, 23,* 335-338.

Everly, C. (1990, January 29). *Personality.* Lecture presented in a graduate course, HLTH 650: Health Problems in Guidance, at the University of Maryland at College Park.

Gleave, G. M. (1960). Legal aspects of medical records. *American Journal of Occupational Therapy, 14,* 180-182.

Hansen, R. (1988). Nationally speaking—Ethics is the issue. *American Journal of Occupational Therapy, 42,* 279-281.

Hansen, R., Kamp, L., & Reitz, S. (1988). Two practitioners' analyses of occupational therapy practice dilemmas. *American Journal of Occupational Therapy, 42,* 312-319.

Kyler-Hutchison, P. (1988). Ethical reasoning and informed consent in occupational therapy. *American Journal of Occupational Therapy, 42,* 283-287.

Overs, R. (1964). Writing work evaluation reports: Core or challenge. *American Journal of Occupational Therapy, 18,* 63-65.

Occupational Therapy Code of Ethics

The American Occupational Therapy Association and its component members are committed to furthering people's ability to function fully within their total environment. To this end the occupational therapist renders service to clients in all stages of health and illness, to institutions, to other professionals and colleagues, to students, and to the general public.

In furthering this commitment, the American Occupational Therapy Association has established the Occupational Therapy Code of Ethics. This Code is intended to be used as a guide to promoting and maintaining the highest standards of ethical behavior.

This Code of Ethics shall apply to all occupational therapy personnel. The term *occupational therapy personnel* shall include individuals who are registered occupational therapists, certified occupational therapy assistants, and occupational therapy students. The roles of practitioner, educator, manager, researcher, and consultant are assumed.

Principle 1 (Beneficence/autonomy)

Occupational therapy personnel shall demonstrate a concern for the welfare and dignity of the recipient of their services.

A. The individual is responsible for providing services without regard to race, creed, national origin, sex, age, handicap, disease entity, social status, financial status or religious affiliation.

B. The individual shall inform those people served of the nature and potential outcomes of treatment and shall respect the right of potential recipients of service to refuse treatment.

C. The individual shall inform subjects involved in education or research activities of the potential outcome of those activities.

D. The individual shall include those people served in the treatment planning process.

E. The individual shall maintain goal-directed and objective relationships with all people served.

F. The individual shall protect the confidential nature of information gained from educational, practice, and investigational activities unless sharing such information could be deemed necessary to protect the well-being of a third party.

G. The individual shall take all reasonable precautions to avoid harm to the recipient of services or detriment to the recipient's property.

H. The individual shall establish fees, based on cost analysis, that are commensurate with services rendered.

Principle 2 (Competence)

Occupational therapy personnel shall actively maintain high standards of professional competence.

A. The individual shall hold the appropriate credential for providing service.

B. The individual shall recognize the need for competence and shall participate in continuing professional development.

C. The individual shall function within the parameters of his or her competence and the standards of the profession.

D. The individual shall refer clients to other service providers or consult with other service providers when additional knowledge and expertise is required.

Principle 3 (Compliance with Laws and Regulations)

Occupational therapy personnel shall comply with laws and Association policies guiding the profession of occupational therapy.

A. The individual shall be acquainted with applicable local, state, federal, and institutional rules and Association policies and shall function accordingly.

B. The individual shall inform employers, employees, and colleagues about those laws and policies that apply to the profession of occupational therapy.

C. The individual shall require those whom they supervise to adhere to the Code of Ethics.

D. The individual shall accurately record and report information.

Principle 4 (Public Information)

Occupational therapy personnel shall provide accurate information concerning occupational therapy services.

A. The individual shall accurately represent his or her competence and training.

B. The individual shall not use or participate in the use of any form of communication that contains a false, fraudulent, deceptive, or unfair statement or claim.

Principle 5 (Professional Relationships)

Occupational therapy personnel shall function with discretion and integrity in relations with colleagues and other professionals, and shall be concerned with the quality of their services.

A. The individual shall report illegal, incompetent, and/or unethical practice to the appropriate authority.

B. The individual shall not disclose privileged information when participating in reviews of peers, programs, or systems.

C. The individual who employs or supervises colleagues shall provide appropriate supervision, as defined in AOTA guidelines or state laws, regulations, and institutional policies.

D. The individual shall recognize the contributions of colleagues when disseminating professional information.

Principle 6 (Professional Conduct)

Occupational therapy personnel shall not engage in any form of conduct that constitutes a conflict of interest or that adversely reflects on the profession.

Enforcement procedures are available from the Department of Professional Services, 1383 Piccard Drive, Rockville, MD 20850. Complaints should be addressed to the Standards and Ethics Chair at the same address.

Approved by the Representative Assembly, April 1988.

This document replaces the Principles of Occupational Therapy Ethics, originally approved, April 1977 and approved as revised, 1979.

Previously published and copyrighted in 1988 by the American Occupational Therapy Association in the *American Journal of Occupational Therapy, 42,* 795-796.

Enforcement Procedure for
Occupational Therapy Code of Ethics

A. PREAMBLE

The American Occupational Therapy Association has developed the Occupational Therapy Code of Ethics in the exercise of its responsibility for promoting quality standards of professional conduct in the practice of occupational therapy. This Code applies directly to all individual members of the Association. The Association further encourages recognition of this Code by all other individuals, organizations, and institutions involved with the profession.

To ensure maintenance of this Code and compliance by Association members, procedures have been developed for the investigation and adjudication of alleged violations. These procedures are intended to enable the Association to act fairly in the performance of its responsibilities as a professional organization. Their purpose is also to safeguard the rights of individuals against whom complaints have been made.

As preamble to the official procedures, the Association urges particular attention to the following issues:

Professional Responsibility—All practitioners of occupational therapy have an obligation to maintain standards of ethics in the practice of their profession and to promote and support these same standards among their colleagues. Each therapist must be alert to practices which undermine these standards and be obligated to take whatever remedial action is required. At the same time, therapists must carefully weigh their judgments of unethical practice to ensure that they are based on objective evaluation and not on personal bias or prejudice.

Confidentiality—Strict confidentiality shall be maintained by all who are involved in the reporting, monitoring, and enforcing of alleged infractions of the Occupational Therapy Code of Ethics. Special care must be exercised at the preliminary review and investigation stages. The maintenance of confidentiality, however, shall not interfere with the provision of proper notice to all parties with an interest in the disciplinary proceedings. Likewise, final decisions of the Judicial Council and the Appeals Panel will be publicized as described in these procedures.

Rules of Evidence—Formal rules of evidence which are employed in legal proceedings do not apply to these "Procedures for Disciplinary Action." The Judicial Council and the Appeals Panel can consider any evidence which they deem appropriate and pertinent. In general, appeals cases shall be limited to the proceedings before the Judicial Council, although the Panel may consider additional evidence, if in its opinion further evidence is required to ensure a fair decision.

Advisory Opinions—On its own initiative, or at the request of others, the Standards and Ethics Commission may issue advisory opinions on the interpretation and application of the Occupational Therapy Code of Ethics. All advisory opinions shall be in writing and signed by the Chair of the Standards and Ethics Commission. Advisory opinions shall be subject to subsequent review and approval by the Representative Assembly.

Jurisdiction—The American Occupational Therapy Association shall have jurisdiction in the monitoring and enforcement of the Occupational Therapy Code of Ethics over all members of the Association.

B. Disciplinary Procedures

1. Complaint

Complaints stating an alleged violation of the Association's Occupational Therapy Code of Ethics may originate from any individual or group within or outside the Association. All complaints must be in writing, signed by the complainant(s), and submitted to the Chair of the Standards and Ethics Commission at the address of the Association's National Office. All complaints shall be timely and shall identify the person against whom the complaint is directed, the actions which occasion the complaint, and the ethical principles which the complainants believe have been violated.

2. Investigation

Within 90 days of receipt of a complaint the Standards and Ethics Commission (SEC) shall make a preliminary assessment of the complaint and decide whether a formal investigation is warranted.

If a formal investigation is required, the SEC shall appoint an Investigation Committee, composed of one or more members of the Association. Within 15 days of its appointment this Committee shall notify the individual against whom the complaint has been made that an investigation is being conducted. This notification shall include a description of the complaint and an explanation of the alleged violation. The individual charged in the complaint shall be given 30 days from receipt of the notification to respond in writing to the Committee.

The Committee may conduct a hearing if both the complainant and the individual against whom the complaint is directed are present. The individual charged in the complaint must be given full opportunity to refute all charges. Apart from the complainant and the charged party, no other persons will participate in, or attend, the hearing without prior approval of the Committee. Fifteen days in advance of the hearing the Committee will notify all participants of the date, time, and place for the hearing.

Within 90 days of its appointment the Committee shall report to the SEC. The Committee's report shall state its findings regarding the validity of the complaint and the need for a formal charge of violation of the Association's ethical standards.

3. Standards and Ethics Commission Review and Decision

The Standards and Ethics Commission shall review the Investigation Committee's report and decide within 60 days of receipt of the report whether a formal charge by the Association is warranted. The SEC may, in the conduct of its review, take whatever further investigatory actions it deems necessary.

If the SEC decides that a formal charge is warranted, the President of the Association shall be so notified and a Judicial Council shall be established.

At this time all parties to the complaint shall be notified in writing of the SEC decision. This notification shall include a statement of the formal charge and a rationale for the decision.

4. The Judicial Council

The Judicial Council, comprised of three members in good standing of the Association, shall be appointed by the President of the Association within 30 days of the notification to hear the formal charges against the individual and decide on the merits of the case.

Thirty days in advance of the hearing, the Judicial Council shall notify in writing all parties of the date, time, and place for the hearing. Within 20 days of notification of the hearings, the individual charged by the Association may submit to the Council a response to the Association's charges.

Legal counsel shall represent the Association at the hearing.

The individual charged may be represented by legal counsel. Full opportunity to refute all charges shall be afforded. All parties shall have the opportunity to confront and cross-examine witnesses. Testimony may be presented by others than those who are parties to the charge. A record of the hearing shall be made.

Within 15 days after the hearing, the Judicial Council shall notify the President of the Association of its decision, which shall include whatever disciplinary action might be required. Disciplinary action for members of the Association shall be limited to censure, suspension, or expulsion from the Association.

Within 15 days of notice from the Judicial Council, the President, on behalf of the Association, shall notify all parties, and the original complainant, of the Council's decision. The President shall notify appropriate bodies within the Association. The President shall also make whatever further notifications are required for the benefit of the individual charged, the Association, and/or the general public.

5. Appeal Process

Within 30 days after the notification of the Council's decision any individual or individuals judged deserving of disciplinary action may appeal the judgment to the Executive Board of the Association. This appeal shall be written, signed by the appealing party, and delivered to the Executive Director at the Association's National Office. The basis for the appeal shall be fully explained in this document.

The appeal must related to issues and procedures that are part of the record of the hearing before the Judicial Council. The appeal may also address the substance of the disciplinary action.

The Association shall be given 15 days after receipt of the appeal to respond in writing to the Appeals Panel.

The Vice-President, Secretary, and Treasurer of the Association shall constitute the Appeals Panel. In the event of vacancies in these positions or the existence of a potential conflict of interest, the President shall appoint replacements drawn from among the other Board members. The President shall not serve on the Appeals Panel.

Within 45 days after the appeal is received, the Panel shall determine whether a hearing is required. If the Panel decides that a hearing is necessary, timely notice for such hearing shall be given to the appealing party. Participants at the hearing shall be limited to the appealing party and legal counsel (if so desired), legal counsel for the Association, and any others approved in advance by the Appeals Panel.

Within 45 days after receipt of the appeal, if there is no hearing, or within 15 days after the appeals hearing, the Appeals Panel shall notify the President of the Association of its decision. The President shall immediately notify the appealing party.

For Association purposes, the decision of the Appeals Panel shall be final.

6. Notification
All notification referred to in this procedure shall be in writing and shall be by certified, return-receipt mail.

7. Records and Reports
At the completion of this procedure all records and reports shall be returned to the Chair of the Standards and Ethics Commission. The original records and reports shall be filed in the confidential file of the Executive Director of the Association. All other copies shall be destroyed.

AOTA:SEC:dd
11/15/88

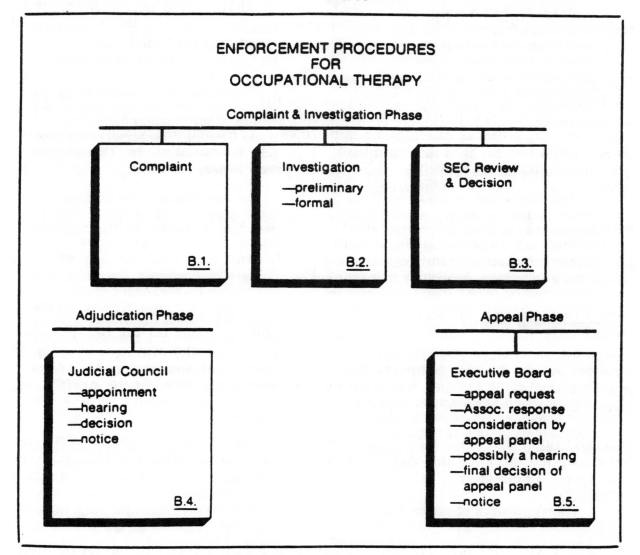

AOTCB

AMERICAN OCCUPATIONAL THERAPY CERTIFICATION BOARD, INC. PROCEDURES FOR DISCIPLINARY ACTION

SECTION A. <u>Preamble</u>

In exercising its responsibility for promoting and maintaining standards of professional conduct in the practice of occupational therapy, the American Occupational Therapy Certification Board, Inc ("AOTCB") has adopted these procedures for the investigation and adjudication of complaints concerning persons who have been certified by the AOTCB as Occupational Therapists, Registered, Certified Occupational Therapy Assistants, or who have applied for such certification. These procedures are intended to enable the AOTCB, through its Disciplinary Action Committee ("DAC"), to act fairly in the performance of its responsibilities to the public as a certifying agency, and to ensure that the rights of individuals against whom complaints have been made are protected.

<u>The purpose of the disciplinary action program</u> - The central purpose of the AOTCB's disciplinary action program is the protection of the public from those practitioners whose professional performance or fitness to practice reflects incompetence, breaches of ethics, or impairment. The disciplinary action program is not intended to be solely punitive; it is also intended to be rehabilitative, providing insofar as possible incentive to practitioners to engage in the safe, proficient and/or competent practice of occupational therapy.

<u>Rules of Evidence</u> - Formal rules of evidence which are employed in legal proceedings do not apply to disciplinary action proceedings. The AOTCB Disciplinary Action Committee and the Appeals Panel may consider any evidence which they deem appropriate and pertinent.

<u>Advisory Opinion</u> - On its own initiative, or at the request of others, the AOTCB Disciplinary Action Committee may issue advisory opinions on the interpretation and application of the disciplinary program. This is a mechanism for obtaining an opinion before the fact or in relation to a hypothetical situation. All advisory opinions shall be in writing, approved by the Board of Directors of the AOTCB and signed by the President of the AOTCB.

<u>Jurisdiction</u> - The DAC shall have jurisdiction over all who are certified or who have applied to take the AOTCB Certification Examination for Occupational Therapist, Registered ("OTR") or Certified Occupational Therapy Assistant ("COTA").

SECTION B. <u>Grounds for Discipline</u> The grounds for disciplinary action for failure to engage in the safe, proficient and/or competent practice of occupational therapy are:

1. <u>Incompetence</u> — Engaging in conduct which evidences a lack of knowledge of, or lack of ability or failure to apply, the prevailing principles and/or skills of the profession for which the individual has been certified.

2. <u>Unethical Behavior</u> — Violating prevailing ethical standards of the profession relating to the safe, proficient and/or competent practice of occupational therapy, including:

   a. Making false statements or providing false information in connection with an application for certification.

   b. Misrepresenting one's credentials (education, training, experience, competence).

   c. Engaging in false, misleading or deceptive advertising.

   d. Obtaining or attempting to obtain compensation by fraud or deceit.

   e. Violating any federal or state statute or law which relates to the practice for which the individual has a certificate.

   f. Engaging in assault and battery of patients or others with whom the practitioner has a professional relationship.

   g. Engaging in sexual misconduct or abuse involving patients or others with whom the practitioner has a professional relationship.

   h. Being convicted of a crime, the circumstances of which substantially relate to the practice of occupational therapy or indicate an inability to engage in the practice of occupational therapy safely, proficiently and/or competently.

   i. Otherwise violating the prevailing standards of the profession relating to the safe, proficient and/or competent practice of occupational therapy.

3. <u>Impairment</u> — The inability to engage in the practice of occupational therapy safely, proficiently and/or competently as a result of substance abuse, or physical or psychological disability. This includes, but is not limited to:

   a. Engaging in professional practice while one's ability to practice is impaired by alcohol or other drugs.

   b. Engaging in practice while one's ability to practice is impaired by reason of physical or mental disability or disease.

   c. Being adjudicated mentally incompetent by a court.

SECTION C.   Sanctions

The Disciplinary Action Committee may impose any one or more of the following sanctions:

1.   Reprimand, which means a formal expression of disapproval which shall be retained in the certificant's file but shall not be publicly announced.

2.   Censure, which means a formal expression of disapproval which is publicly announced.

3.   Ineligibility for certification, which means that an individual is barred from becoming certified by the AOTCB, either indefinitely or for a certain duration.

4.   Probation, which means continued certification is subject to fulfillment of specified conditions, e.g., monitoring, education, supervision, and/or counseling.

5.   Suspension, which means the loss of certification for a certain duration, after which the individual may be required to apply for reinstatement.

6.   Revocation, which means permanent loss of certification.

SECTION D.   Disciplinary Procedures

1.   Initiation of the Disciplinary Process

        The disciplinary action process shall be initiated upon receipt by the DAC of information that appears to be relevant to an individual's fitness to practice or otherwise constitute grounds for disciplinary action under these procedures. Ordinarily,this will occur when a complaint is received by the DAC from an individual or group; however, the DAC may also commence a disciplinary action process without such a complaint upon receipt of information that indicates that there may be grounds for disciplinary action. For purposes of these procedures, this shall also be considered a complaint.

2.   Investigation

        The Disciplinary Action Committee Staff Administrator ("Administrator") and the Chair of the Disciplinary Action Committee shall make a preliminary assessment of each complaint and decide whether a formal investigation is warranted. The Administrator and the Chair of the DAC have the authority to dismiss frivolous complaints, but any such dismissal shall be reported to the full DAC.

If it is determined by the Administrator and the Chair of the DAC that a formal investigation is warranted, the Administrator shall immediately notify the subject of the complaint of the investigation. This notification shall be in writing and shall include a description of the complaint and the identity of the complainant. The notice shall be sent by certified mail. The subject of the complaint shall have 30 days from the date notification is sent to respond in writing to the complaint. The Administrator may extend this period up to an additional 30 days upon request, provided sufficient justification for the extension is given.

The Administrator shall be responsible for conducting the formal investigation. In discharging this responsibility, he or she may utilize the services of AOTCB staff, counsel and/or independent investigators.

Within 90 days after the notice of investigation is given to the individual charged in the complaint, the Administrator shall provide a written report to the DAC. The report shall state the Administrator's findings regarding the complaint, and shall include the written responses, if any, made by the individual charged in the complaint.

In cases where a state regulatory board has taken disciplinary action against an individual, the Administrator will contact the state regulatory board for information and will include this information in his or her report to the DAC.

Failure to respond or to cooperate in the disciplinary action proceedings shall be sufficient grounds for the imposition of sanctions by the DAC.

If at any point, the subject of a complaint requests that his or her certification or application to take the examination be withdrawn, the disciplinary action procedure may be dismissed within the discretion of the DAC; however, public notice of the withdrawal may be given.

3. Disciplinary Action Committee Review and Decision

The DAC shall review the report of the Administrator and, based upon the available information, either (a) dismiss the complaint; (b) direct the Administrator to obtain additional information; (c) stay the proceedings pending completion of any disciplinary action proceedings by a state regulatory board or; (d) make a preliminary determination of disciplinary action. If the DAC makes a preliminary determination of disciplinary action, it shall also schedule a hearing.

The Administrator shall give the subject of the complaint written notice of the DAC's action. If the DAC has made a preliminary determination of disciplinary action, the notice shall state the grounds for the preliminary determination, the proposed sanction and the time, date and place of the scheduled hearing.

The subject of the complaint may waive his or her right to a hearing by accepting the DAC's preliminary determination of disciplinary action and proposed sanction. If the subject of the complaint does not accept the preliminary determination of the disciplinary action and proposed sanction, there shall be a hearing on the compliant before the DAC as scheduled. The subject of the complaint shall be solely responsible for all of his/her own expenses related to the hearing.

Apart from the complainant,the subject of the complaint and his or her legal counsel, the Administrator, the DAC, and the counsel for the AOTCB, no other persons may participate in, or attend, the hearing without forty-eight (48) hours prior written notice to the DAC.

Following the hearing, the DAC shall notify in writing all parties to the complaint of its decision.

If an individual's certification is suspended or revoked, or he or she is placed on probation or censured, all occupational therapy state regulatory boards and occupational therapy state associations will be notified and an announcement will be included in one or more publications of general circulation to persons engaged or otherwise interested in the profession of occupational therapy. The AOTCB may also disclose the disciplinary action to persons inquiring about the status of an individual's certification, including, but not limited to, state regulatory boards, employers, insurers and the general public.

4. Appeal Process

Within thirty (30) days after the notification of the DAC's decision, any individual or individuals judged deserving of disciplinary action may appeal the judgment to the Board of Directors of the AOTCB. A notice of appeal, which must be in writing and signed by the appealing party, shall be sent by the appealing party to the Board of Directors of the AOTCB in care of the Executive Director. The basis for the appeal shall be fully explained in this notice.

The AOTCB Board of Directors shall have 30 days after receipt of the notice of appeal to form an Appeals Panel.

Three members of the AOTCB Board of Directors shall constitute the Appeals Panel. The President shall not serve on the Appeals Panel.

The appeal must relate to evidence, issues and procedures that are part of the record of the DAC hearing and decision. The appeal may also address the substance of the disciplinary action. However, the Panel may consider additional evidence if, in its opinion, consideration of such evidence is required to ensure a fair decision.

Within 15 days after the notice of appeal is received by the Appeals Panel, the Panel shall determine whether a hearing is required. If the Panel decides that a hearing is necessary, timely notice for such hearings shall be given to the appealing party. Participants at the hearing shall be limited to the appealing party and legal counsel (if so desired), legal counsel for the AOTCB, and any others approved in advance by the Appeals Panel.

Within 15 days after receipt of the notice of appeal, if there is no hearing, or within 15 days after the appeals hearing, the Appeals Panel shall notify the President and the Executive Director of the AOTCB of its decision. The President shall immediately notify the appealing party.

The decision of the Appeals Panel shall be final.

5. <u>Notification</u>

All notifications referred to in these procedures shall be in writing and shall be by certified, return receipt mail unless otherwise indicated.

6. <u>Records and Reports</u>

At the completion of this procedure, all records and reports shall be returned to the Administrator. The complete files in the disciplinary proceedings shall be carefully reviewed and everything discarded except information on the initial basis for the challenge, the actual evidence in resolving the proceeding, and the disposition of the case.

Revised: June 1989
Revised: October 1989
Revised: August 1991

/sm

Appendices

The following appendices provide supplementary material relevant to the subject of documentation and documentation review. All four appendices reprint material taken from the Medicare guidelines, published by the Health Care Financing Administration.

- *Appendix A on page 244 covers the medical review of part B intermediary outpatient occupational therapy bills.*

- *Appendix B on page 256 deals with Medicare coverage and limitations.*

- *Appendix C on page 262 covers the medical review of part B intermediary outpatient speech-language pathology bills.*

- *Appendix D on page 277 covers the medical review of part B intermediary outpatient physical therapy bills.*

3906.   MEDICAL REVIEW (MR) OF PART B INTERMEDIARY OUTPATIENT OCCUPATIONAL THERAPY (OT) BILLS

These guidelines assist the reviewer in understanding the field of OT as well as facilitate the MR process. They are flexible and neither guarantee a minimum amount of coverage nor establish a maximum coverage amount. They do not cover all situations. They are intended to use in conjunction with §3100 and the knowledge of medical and occupational therapy consultants. If possible, have occupational therapists review OT bills.

Medically review all outpatient OT claims referred to Level II or III, regardless of the setting.

Claims Documentation - medically review each claim referred to Level II or III for outpatient OT services to make a coverage determination. The following provider documentation is required:

    o   <u>Facility and Patient Identification</u> - (Facility name, patient's name, provider number, HICN, age).

    o   <u>Physician Referral and Date.</u>

    o   <u>Date of Last Certification</u> - The date on which the plan of treatment was last certified by the physician.

    o   <u>Diagnosis</u> - The primary diagnosis for which OT services were rendered is listed first; other diagnoses applicable to the patient or that influence care follow.

    o   <u>Duration</u> - The length of time OT services have been rendered (in days) from the date services were initiated for the diagnosis at the billing provider (including the last day in the current billing period).

    o   <u>Number of Visits</u> - The number of patient visits completed since OT services were initiated by the billing provider for the diagnosis being treated. The total visits to date (including the last visit in the billing period) is given rather than for each separate billing.

    o   <u>Date of Onset</u> (Occurrence Code 11) - The date of onset of the primary OT diagnosis for which OT services were rendered by the billing provider.

    o   <u>Date Treatment Started</u> (Occurrence Code 35) - The date OT services were initiated by the billing provider for the primary OT diagnosis being treated.

o   Billing Period - When OT services began and ended in the billing period (from-through dates).

o   Medical History - The provider submits the medical history pertinent to, or which influences, the OT treatment, including a brief description of the functional status of the patient prior to the onset of the condition requiring OT and pertinent prior OT treatment.

o   OT Initial Evaluation and Date. (At the billing provider.)

o   Plan of Treatment and Date Established.

o   OT Progress Notes - The provider supplies updated status reports concerning the patient's current functional abilities/limitations.

1.   Medical History.--If a history of previous OT treatment is not available, the provider provides a general summary regarding the patient's past relevent medical history recorded during the initial evaluation with the patient/family or through contact with the referring physician. Information regarding prior OT treatment for the current condition, progress made, and treatment by the referring physician is provided when available. The level of function prior to the current exacerbation or onset is described.

The patient's medical history, as it relates to OT, includes the date of onset and/or exacerbation of the illness or injury. If the patient has had prior therapy for the same condition, use that history in conjunction with the patient's current assessment to establish whether additional treatment is reasonable.

The history of treatments from a previous provider is necessary for patients who have transferred to a new provider. For example, if surgery has been performed, obtain the type and date. The date of onset and type of surgical procedure should be specific for diagnoses such as fractures. For other diagnoses, such as arthritis, the date of onset may be general. Establish it from the date the patient first required medical treatment. For other types of chronic diagnoses, the history gives the date of the change or deterioration in the patient's condition and a description of the changes that necessitate skilled OT.

2.   Evaluation.--Approve an OT initial evaluation, (excluding routine screening) when it is reasonable and necessary for the therapist to determine if there is an expectation that either restorative or maintenance services are appropriate. Approve reevaluations when the patient exhibits a demonstrable change in physical functional ability, to reestablish appropriate treatment goals, or when required for ongoing assessment of the patient's rehabilitation needs. Approve initial evaluations or reevaluations that are reasonable and necessary based on the patient's condition, even though the expectations are not realized, or when the evaluation determines that skilled rehabilitation is not needed.

The OT evaluation establishes the physical and cognitive baseline data necessary for assessing expected rehabilitation potential, setting realistic goals, and measuring progress. The evaluation of the patient's functional deficits and level of assistance needed forms the basis for the OT treatment goals. Objective tests and measurements are used (when possible) to establish base-line data.

The provider documents the patient's functional loss and the level of assistance requiring skilled OT intervention resulting from conditions such as:

     o   <u>Activities of Daily Living (ADL) Dependence</u> - The individual is dependent upon skilled intervention for performance of activities of daily living. These include, but are not limited to, signficant physical and/or cognitive functional loss, or loss of previous functional gains in the ability to:

          -- Feed, eat, drink;
          -- Bathe;
          -- Dress;
          -- Perform personal hygiene;
          -- Groom; or
          -- Perform toileting.

This could include management and care of orthoses and/or other adaptive equipment, or other customized therapeutic adaptations.

     o   <u>Functional Limitation</u> - The individual is dependent upon skilled OT intervention in functional training, observation, assessment, and environmental adaptation due to, but not limited to:

          -- Lack of awareness of sensory cues, or safety hazards;
          -- Impaired attention span;
          -- Impaired strength;
          -- Incoordination;
          -- Abnormal muscle tone;
          -- Range of motion limitations;
          -- Impaired body scheme;
          -- Perceptual deficits;
          -- Impaired balance/head control; and
          -- Environmental barriers.

     o   <u>Safety Dependence/Secondary Complications</u> - A safety problem exists when a patient, without skilled OT intervention, cannot handle him/herself in a manner that is physically and/or cognitively safe. This may extend to daily living or to acquired secondary complications which could potentially intensify medical sequelae such as fracture nonunion, or skin breakdown. Safety dependence may be demonstrated by high probability of falling, lack of environmental safety awareness, swallowing difficulties, abnormal agressive/destructive behavior, severe pain, loss of skin sensation, progressive joint contracture, and joint protection/preservation requiring skilled OT intervention to protect the patient from further medical complication.

If the goal for the patient is to increase functional abilities and decrease the level of assistance needed, the initial evaluation must measure the patient's starting functional abilities and level of assistance required.

3. <u>Plan of Treatment</u>.--The OT plan of treatment must include specific functional goals and a reasonable estimate of when they will be reached (e.g., 6 weeks). It is not adequate to estimate "1 to 2 months on an ongoing basis." The plan must include specific OT procedures, frequency, and duration of treatment. The provider submits changes in the plan with the progress notes.

The plan of treatment contains:

o   <u>Type of OT Procedures</u> - Describes the specific nature of the therapy to be provided.

o   <u>Frequency of Visits</u> - An estimate of the frequency of treatment to be rendered (e.g., 3x week).

The provider's medical documentation should justify the intensity of services rendered. This is crucial when the treatments are given more frequently than 3 times a week.

o   <u>Estimated Duration</u> - Identifies the length of time over which the services are to be rendered. It may be expressed in days, weeks, or months.

o   <u>Diagnoses</u> - Includes the OT diagnosis if different from the medical diagnosis. The OT diagnosis should be based on objective tests, whenever possible.

o   <u>Functional OT Goals (short or long-term)</u> - Reflects the occupational therapist's and/or physician's description of what functional physical/cognitive abilities the patient is expected to achieve.

Assume that certain factors may change or influence the level of achievement. If this occurs, the occupational therapist explains the factors which led to the change in functional goal(s).

o   <u>Rehabilitation Potential</u> - The occupational therapist's and/or physician's expectation concerning the patient's ability to meet the established goals.

4. <u>Progress Reports (Treatment Summary for Billing Period)</u>.--The provider documents and reports:

o   The initial functional status of the patient;

o   The patient's functional status and progress (or lack of progress) specific for this reporting period; including clinical findings (amount of physical and/or cognitive assistance needed, range of motion, muscle strength, unaffected limb measurements, etc.); and

o   The patient's expected rehabilitation potential.

10-122   Rev.1424

Where a valid expectation of improvement exists at the time OT services are initiated, or thereafter, the services are covered even though the expectation may not be realized. However, in such instances, the OT services are covered only to the time that no further significant practical improvement can be expected. Progress reports or status summaries must document a continued expectation that the patient's condition will continue to improve significantly in a reasonable and generally predictable period of time.

"Significant," means a generally measurable and substantial increase in the patient's present level of functional independence and competence, compared to that when treatment was initiated. Do not interpret the term "significant" so stringently that you deny a claim simply because of a temporary setback in the patient's progress. For example, a patient may experience an intervening medical complication or a brief period when lack of progress occurs. The medical reviewer may approve the claim if there is still a reasonable expectation that significant improvement in the patient's <u>overall safety</u> <u>or functional ability</u> will occur. However, the provider should document such lack of progress and briefly explain the need for continued skilled OT intervention.

The provider must provide treatment information regarding the status of the patient during the billing period. The provider's progress notes and any needed reevaluation(s) must update the baseline information provided at the initial evaluation. If there is a change in the plan of treatment, it must be documented. Additionally, when a patient is continued from one billing period to another, the progress report(s) must reflect the comparisons between the patient's current functional status and that during the previous billing and/or initial evaluation.

Conduct MR of claims with an understanding that skilled intervention may be needed, and improvement in a patient's condition may occur, even where a patient's full or partial recovery is <u>not</u> possible. For example, a terminally ill patient may begin to exhibit ADL, mobility and/or safety dependence requiring OT services. The fact that full or partial recovery is not possible or rehabilitation potential is not present, does not affect MR coverage decisions. The deciding factor is whether the services are considered reasonable, effective, treatment for the patient's condition and they require the skills of an occupational therapist, or whether they can be safely and effectively carried out by nonskilled personnel, without the occupational therapist's supervision. The reasons for OT must be clear to you, as well as their goals, prior to a favorable coverage determination. They often require review at Level III.

It is essential that the provider documents the updated status in a clear, concise, and objective manner. Objective tests and measurements are stressed when these are practical. The occupational therapist selects the appropriate method to demonstrate current patient status. However, the method chosen, as well as the measures used, should be consistent during the treatment duration. If the method used to demonstrate progress is changed, the reasons for the change should be documented, including how the new method relates to the old. You must have an overview of the purpose of treatment goals in order to compare the patient's current functional status to that in previous reporting periods.

Rev.1424   10-123

<u>Documentation of the patient's current functional status and level of assistance required</u> <u>compared to previous reporting period(s) is of paramount importance.</u> The deficits in <u>functional ability should be clear.</u> Occupational therapists must document functional improvements (or lack thereof) as a result of their treatments. Documentation of functional progress must be stated whenever possible in objective, measurable terms. The following illustrates these principles and demonstrates that significant changes may occur in one or more of these assistance levels:

       a. <u>Change in Level of Assistance.</u>--Occupational therapist's document assistance levels by describing the relationship between functional activities and the need for assistance. Within the assistance levels of minimum, moderate, and maximum, there are intermediate gradations of improvement based on changes in behavior and response to assistance. <u>Improvements at each level must be documented.</u> Documentation should compare the current cognitive and physicial level achieved to that achieved previously. While the need for cognitive assistance often is the more severe and persistent disability, the requirement of physical assistance often is the major obstacle to successful outcomes and subsequent discharge. Interpret the levels as follows:

       o   <u>Total Assistance</u> is the need for 100 percent assistance by one or more persons to perform all physical activities and/or cognitive assistance to elicit a functional response to an external stimulation.

A patient requires total assistance if the documentation indicates the patient is only able to initiate minimal voluntary motor actions and requires the skill of an occupational therapist to develop a therapeutic program or implement a maintenance program to prevent or minimize deterioration.

A cognitively impaired patient requires total assistance when documentation shows external stimuli are required to elicit automatic actions such as swallowing or responding to auditory stimuli. Skills of an occupational therapist are needed to identify and apply strategies for eliciting appropriate, consistent automatic responses to external stimuli.

       o   <u>Maximum Assistance</u> is the need for 75 percent assistance by one person to physicially perform any part of a functional activity and/or cognitive assistance to perform gross motor actions in response to direction.

A patient requires maximum assistance if maximum OT physical support and proprioceptive stimulation is needed for performance of each step of a functional activity, every time it is performed.

A cognitively impaired patient, at this level, may need proprioceptive stimulation and/or one-to-one demonstration by the occupational therapist due to the patient's lack of cognitive awareness of other people or objects in the environment.

       o   <u>Moderate Assistance</u> is the need for 50 percent assistance by one person to perform physical activities or constant cognitive assistance to sustain/complete simple, repetitive activities safely.

A physically impaired patient requires moderate assistance if documentation indicates that moderate OT physical support and proprioceptive stimulation is needed for the patient to perform a functional activity, every time it is performed.

The records submitted should state how a cognitively impaired patient, at this level, requires intermittent one-to-one demonstration or intermittent cueing (physical or verbal) throughout performance of the activity. Moderate assistance is needed when the occupational therapist/caregiver needs to be in the immediate environment to progress the patient through a sequence to complete a functional activity. This level of assistance is required to halt continued repetition of a task and to prevent unsafe, erratic or unpredictable actions that interfere with appropriate sequencing.

         o   Minimum Assistance is the need for 25 percent assistance by one person for physical activities and/or periodic, cognitive assistance to perform functional activities safely.

A physically impaired patient requires minimum assistance if documentation indicates that activities can only be performed after physical set-up by the occupational therapist or caregiver, and if physical help is needed to initiate, or sustain an activity. A review of alternate procedures, sequences and methods may be required.

A cognitively impaired patient requires minimal assistance if documentation indicates help is needed in performing known activities to correct repeated mistakes, to check for compliance with established safety procedures, or to solve problems posed by unexpected hazards.

         o   Standby Assistance is the need for supervision by one person for the patient to perform new activity procedures which were adapted by the therapist for safe and effective performance.

A patient requires standby assistance when errors and the need for safety precautions are not always anticipated by the patient.

         o   Independent Status means that no physical or cognitive assistance is required to perform functional activities.

Patients at this level are able to implement the selected courses of action, consider potential errors and anticipate safety hazards in familiar and new situations.

         b.   Change in Response to Treatment Within Each Level of Assistance.-- Significant improvement must be indicated by documenting a change in one or more of the following categories of patient responses within any level of assistance:

         o   Decreased Refusals. The patient may respond by refusing to attempt performance of an activity because of fear or pain. The documentation should indicate what activity and performance is refused, the reasons, and how the OT plan addresses them.

Rev. 1424   10-125

These responses are often secondary to a change in medical status or medications. If the refusals continue over several days, the therapy program should be put on "hold" until the documentation indicates the refusal response has changed and the patient is willing to attempt performance of functional activities.

For the cognitively impaired patient, refusal to perform can escalate into agressive, destructive or verbally abusive behavior if pressed by the therapist or caregiver to perform. In these cases, a reduction in these behaviors is significant and must be clearly documented, including the skilled OT provided to reduce the abnormal behavior.

For the psychiatrically impaired patient, refusals to participate in an activity frequently are symptoms of the diagnosis. This patient should not be put on a "hold" status due to refusals. If the documentation indicates the patient is receiving OT, contacted regularly, and actively encouraged to participate, medically review the claim to determine if reasonable and necessary skilled care has been rendered.

      o   Increased Consistency. The patient may respond by inconsistently performing functional tasks from day-to-day or within a treatment session.

Approve the claim when the documentation indicates a significant progression in consistency of performance of functional tasks within the same level of assistance.

      o   Increased Generalization. The patient may respond by applying previously learned concepts and performance of one activity to another, similar activity. The records submitted should document a significant increase in scope of activities that the patient can perform, the type of activities, and the skilled OT services rendered.

      c.   A New Skilled Functional Activity is Initiated.--Two examples of skilled care are:

      o   Adding teaching of lower body dressing to a current program of upper body dressing;

      o   Increasing the ability to perform personal hygiene activities for health and social acceptance.

      d.   A New Skilled Compensatory Technique is Added.--(With or without adapted equipment.) Two examples are:

      o   Teaching a patient techniques such as one-handed shoe tying;

      o   Teaching the use of a button hook for buttoning shirt buttons.

      e.   Length of Time in Treatment.--The acceptable length of time in treatment for various disorders is determined by the patient's functional abilities and progress as reflected in the documentation.

10-126   Rev. 1424

5. <u>Level of Complexity of Treatment</u>.--Base decisions on the level of complexity of the services rendered by the occupational therapist and not what the patient is asked to do. Examples of complexity of treatment are:

    a. <u>Skilled OT</u>.--The documentation must indicate that the severity of the physical/emotional/perceptual/cognitive disability requires complex and sophisticated knowledge to identify current and potential capabilities. In addition, consider instructions required by the patient and/or the patient's caregivers. Instructions may be required for activities that most healthy people take for granted. The special knowledge of an occupational therapist is required to decrease or eliminate limitations in functional activity performance imposed by illness or disability. Occupational therapists must often address underlying factors which interfere with the performance of specific activities. Some of these factors could be cognitive, sensory, or perceptual deficits.

The occupational therapist modifies the specific activity by using adapted equipment, making changes in the environment and surrounding objects, altering procedures for accomplishing the task, and providing specialized assistance to meet the patient's current and potential abilities. Skilled services include, but are not limited to reasonable and necessary:

    o   Evaluations of the patient;

    o   Determinations of effective goals and services with the patient and patient's caregivers and other medical professsionals;

    o   Analyzing and modifying functional tasks;

    o   Determinating that the modified task obtains optimum performance through tests and measurements;

    o   Providing instructions of the task(s) to the patient/family/caregivers; and

    o   Periodically reevaluating the patient's status with corresponding readjustment of the OT program.

A period of practice may be approved for the patient and/or patient's caregivers to learn the steps of the task, to verify the task's effectivnesss in improving function, and to check for safe and consistent activity performance.

    b. <u>Nonskilled OT</u>.--When the documentation indicates a patient has attained the therapy goals or has reached the point where no further significant improvement can be expected, the skills of an occupational therapist are not required to <u>maintain function</u> at the level to which it has been restored. Examples of maintenance procedures are:

    o   Daily feeding programs after the adapted procedures are in place;

    o   Routine exercise and strengthing programs;

    o   The practice of coordination and self-care skills on a daily basis; and

    o   Presenting information on energy conservation or pacing, but not having the patient perform the activity.

Rev. 1424   10-127

You may approve a claim because the patient requires the judgment and skills of the occupational therapist to design a safe and effective maintenance program and make <u>periodic</u> checks of its effectiveness. The services of an occupational therapist in <u>carrying out</u> the established maintenance program are not considered reasonable and necessary for the treatment of illness or injury and may not be approved.

      6.   <u>Reporting on New Episode or Condition.</u>--Occasionally, a patient who is receiving or who has received OT services, experiences a new illness. The provider must document the significance of any change to the patient's functional capabilities. This may be by pre and post episodic through nursing notes or physician reports. If the patient is receiving treatment, it might be lengthened. If the patient has completed treatment for the functional deficit; a significant change in the patient's functional status must be documented which warrants a new treatment plan.

3906.1   <u>Other MR Considerations.</u>--

    A. <u>Pain.</u>--Documentation describing the presence or absence of pain and its effect on the patient's functional abilities must be considered in MR decisions. A description of its intensity, type, changing pattern, and location at specific joint ranges of motion materially aids correct MR decisions. Documentation should describe the limitations placed upon the patient's ADL, mobility and/or safety, as well as the subjective progress made in the reduction of pain through treatment.

    B. <u>Therapeutic Programs.</u>--The objective documentation should support the skilled nature of the program, and/or the need for the design and establishment of a maintenance OT program. The goals should generally be to increase functional abilities in ADL, mobility or patient safety. Documentation should indicate the goals and type of program provided.

Approve claims when the therapeutic program, because of documented medical complications, the condition of the patient, or complexity of the OT employed, must be rendered by, or under, the supervision of an occupational therapist. For example, while functional ADL may often be performed safely and effectively by nonskilled personnel, the presence of fracture nonunion, severe joint pain, or other medical or safety complications may warrant skilled occupational therapist intervention to render the service and/or to establish a safe maintenance program. In these cases, the complications and the skilled services, they require, must be documented by physician orders and/or occupational therapist notes. To make correct MR decisions, the patient's losses and/or dependencies in ADL, mobility and safety must be documented. The possibility of adverse effects from the improper performance of an otherwise unskilled service does not make it a skilled service unless there is documentation to support why skilled OT is needed for the patient's medical condition and/or safety.

Approve establishment and design of a maintenance exercise program to fit the patient's level of ADL, function, and any instructions supportive personnel and/or family members need to safely and effectively carry it out. Reevaluation may be approved when reasonable and necessary to readjust the maintenance program to meet the changing needs of the patient. There must be adequate justification for readjusting a maintenance program, e.g., loss of previous functional gains.

C. Cardiac Rehabilitation Exercise.--Occupational therapy is not covered when furnished in connection with cardiac rehabilitation exercise program services (see Coverage Issues Manual 35-25) unless there is also a diagnosed noncardiac condition requiring it e.g., where a patient who is recuperating from an acute phase of heart disease may have had a stroke which requires OT. (While the cardiac rehabilitation exercise program may be considered by some a form of OT, it is a specialized program conducted and/or supervised by specially trained personnel whose services are performed under the direct supervision of a physician.)

D. Transfer Training.--The documentation should describe the patient's functional limitations in transfer ability that warrant skilled OT intervention. Documentation should include the special transfer training needed to perform functional daily living skills and any training needed by supportive personnel and/or family members to safely and effectively carry it out. Approve transfer training when the documentation supports a skilled need for evaluation, design and effective monitoring and instruction of the special transfer technique for safety and completion of the functional activities of daily living or mobility task.

Documentation that supports only repetitious carrying out of the transfer method, once established, and monitored for safety and completion is noncovered care.

E. Fabrication of and Training in Use of Orthoses Prostheses and Adaptive Equipment.--Approve reasonable and necessary fabrication of orthoses, prostheses, adaptive equipment, and any reasonable and necessary skilled training needed in their safe and effective use. The documentation must indicate the need for the device and training required.

F. OT Forms.--Documentation may be submitted on a specific form or may be copies of the provider's record. You may require a specific form if you find it more efficient than using provider records; however, it must capture the needed MR information. If you choose to require a particular form, show the OMB clearance number. The information must be complete. If it is not, return the bill for the additional information and request the missing information. The information you require to review the bill is that required by an occupational therapist to properly treat a patient.

G. Certification and Recertification.--OT services must be certified and recertified by a physician. They must be furnished while the patient is under the care of a physician. They must be furnished under a written plan of treatment established by the physician or a qualified occupational therapist providing such services. If the plan is established by a occupational therapist, it must be reviewed periodically by the physician. The plan of care must be established (reduced to writing by either professional or the provider when it makes a written record of the oral orders) before treatment is begun. When outpatient OT services are continued under the same plan of treatment for a period of time, the physician must certify at intervals of at least every 30 days that there is a continuing need for such services. Obtain the recertification when reviewing the plan of treatment since the same interval of at least 30 days is required for the review of the plans. Recertification must be signed by the physician who reviewed the plan of treatment. Any changes to the treatment plan established by the occupational therapist must be in writing and signed by the occupational therapist or by the attending physician. The physician may change a plan of treatment established by the occupational therapist, the occupational therapist may not alter a plan of treatment established by a physician.

3906.2   <u>Occupational Therapy Availability</u>.--There may be instances where two or more disciplines are providing therapy services to the same patient. There may also be occasions where these services are duplicative. In many instances, however, the description of the services appears duplicative, but the documentation proves that they are not. Some examples where there is <u>not</u> a duplication:

o   <u>Transfers</u> - Physical therapy instructs the patient in transfers to ascertain the level of safety with the techniques. Occupational therapy instructs and utilizes transfers as they relate to the performance of daily living skills, i.e., transfer from wheelchair to bathtub to bathe.

o   <u>Pulmonary</u> - Physical therapy teaches the patient an adapted breathing program. Occupational therapy carries the breathing retraining program into activities of daily living training.

o   <u>Hip Fractures/Arthroplasties</u> - Physical therapy instructs the patient in hip precautions and gait training. Occupational therapy carries out and reinforces the precautions when training the patient in activities of daily living, e.g., lower extremity dressing, toileting, and bathing.

o   <u>CVA</u> - Physical therapy utilizes upper extremity neurodevelopmental (NDT) techniques to assist the patient in positioning the upper extremities on a walker and in gait training. Occupational therapy utilizes upper extremity neurodevelopmental (NDT) techniques to increase the functional use of the upper extremity for dressing, bathing, grooming, etc.

medicare
Carriers Manual
Part 3 – Claims Process

ADVANCE COPY
OF FINAL ISSUANCE

Department of Health
and Human Services

Health Care Financing
Administration

Transmittal No. 1209   Date   AUGUST 1987

REVISED MATERIAL   REVISED PAGES   REPLACED PAGES

Table of Contents
  Chapter II   2-1 - 2-6 (6 pp.)   2-1 - 2-6 (6 pp.)
Sec. 2200 - 2203   2-87 - 2-88 (2 pp.)   2-87 - 2-88 (2 pp.)
Sec. 2215 - 2220   2-94.1 - 2-94.10 (10 pp.) 2-94.1 - 2-94.4D (8 pp.)
Sec. 2476.4 - 2480   2-141 - 2-142 (2 pp.)   2-141 - 2-142 (2 pp.)
Sec. 6130.2-6130.2(Cont.)   6-31 - 6-32.3 (5 pp.)   6-31 - 6-32.2 (4 pp.)
Sec. 6999   6-55 - 6-56 (2 pp.)   6-55 - 5-56 (2 pp.)
Sec. 6999 (Exhibit 31)   6-107 (1 p.)   6-107 (1 p.)

NEW IMPLEMENTING INSTRUCTIONS—EFFECTIVE DATE: For services furnished on and after July 1, 1987. (Search your records and reopen any previously denied claims submitted by qualified occupational therapists in independent practice for services furnished since July 1, 1987.)

Section 2200, Coverage of Provider Outpatient Physical Therapy and Speech Pathology Services Under Medical Insurance.—Section 9337 of P.L. 99-509, the Omnibus Budget Reconciliation Act of 1986, provides for the coverage of outpatient occupational therapy services under Part B furnished by an independently practicing occupational therapist. A reference to this new coverage has been added.

Section 2215, Services Furnished by a Physical or Occupational Therapist in Independent Practice.—A reference to the outpatient occupational therapy benefit has been added.

Section 2217, Covered Occupational Therapy.—This section implements coverage for outpatient occupational therapy services, in accordance with §9337 of P.L. 99-509.

Section 2480, Limitation on Reimbursement of Services Furnished by a Physical or Occupational Therapist in Independent Practice.—A reference to the new outpatient occupational therapy benefit has been added.

CHANGE IN PROCEDURE — EFFECTIVE DATE: SEPTEMBER 11, 1987

<u>Section 6130.2, Disposition Codes (Columns 19-20)</u> — This section explains the procedure for verifying dates of death (Disposition Code 02). You have 2 options: sending form HCFA-1980 to the Social Security Office, or sending a date of death development letter. If the development letter option is chosen, there is now <u>only one</u> letter that may be used (revised Exhibit 31). <u>Locally approved letters are no longer permitted.</u>

This change is necessary due to beneficiary complaints regarding the content of some of the letters being sent. The use of a standard letter will insure uniformity nationwide.

<u>Section 6999, Exhibit 31</u> — This exhibit is the <u>only</u> development letter to be used in verifying date of death, and replaces the current Exhibit 31, and all other locally approved letters.

    o   Mental retardation with disorders such as aphasia or dysarthria; and

    o   Laryngeal carcinoma requiring laryngectomy resulting in aphonia may warrant therapy of the laryngectomized patient so he can develop new communication skills through esophageal speech and/or use of the electrolarynx.

NOTE: Many patients who do not require speech pathology services as defined above do require services involving nondiagnostic, nontherapeutic, routine, repetitive, and reinforced procedures or services for their general good and welfare; e.g., the practicing of word drills. Such services do not constitute speech pathology services for Medicare purposes and would not be covered since they do not require performance by or the supervision of a qualified speech pathologist.

2217.   COVERED OCCUPATIONAL THERAPY

    A.   <u>General</u>.—Covered occupational therapy services must relate directly and specifically to a written treatment regimen established by the physician, after any needed consultation with the qualified occupational therapist, or by the occupational therapist providing the services.

Occupational therapy is medically prescribed treatment concerned with improving or restoring functions which have been impaired by illness or injury or, where function has been permanently lost or reduced by illness or injury, to improve the individual's ability to perform those tasks required for independent functioning. Such therapy may involve:

    o   The evaluation, and reevaluation as required, of a patient's level of function by administering diagnostic and prognostic tests;

    o   The selection and teaching of task-oriented therapeutic activities designed to restore physical function, e.g., use of woodworking activities on an inclined table to restore shoulder, elbow and wrist range of motion lost as a result of burns;

    o   The planning, implementing, and supervising of individualized therapeutic activity programs as part of an overall "active treatment" program for a patient with a diagnosed psychiatric illness, e.g., the use of sewing activities which require following a pattern to reduce confusion and restore reality orientation in a schizophrenic patient;

    o   The planning and implementing of therapeutic tasks and activities to restore sensory-integrative function, e.g., providing motor and tactile activities to increase sensory input and improve response for a stroke patient with functional loss resulting in a distorted body image;

    o   The teaching of compensatory technique to improve the level of independence in the activities of daily living, for example:

    —   Teaching a patient who has lost the use of an arm how to pare potatoes and chop vegetables with one hand;

    —   Teaching an upper extremity amputee how to functionally utilize a prosthesis;

Rev. 1209   2-94.7

    —   Teaching a stroke patient new techniques to enable him to perform feeding, dressing and other activities as independently as possible; or

    —   Teaching a hip fracture/hip replacement patient techniques of standing tolerance and balance to enable him or her to perform such functional activities as dressing and homemaking tasks.

    o   The designing, fabricating, and fitting of orthotic and self-help devices, e.g., making a hand splint for a patient with rheumatoid arthritis to maintain the hand in a functional position or constructing a device which would enable an individual to hold a utensil and feed himself independently; or

    o   Vocational and prevocational assessment and training, subject to the limitations specified in §2217.B.

Only a qualified occupational therapist has the knowledge, training, and experience required to evaluate and, as necessary, reevaluate a patient's level of function, determine whether an occupational therapy program could reasonably be expected to improve, restore, or compensate for lost function and, where appropriate, recommend to the physician a plan of treatment.

    B.   <u>Coverage Criteria</u>.--Occupational therapy designed to improve function is considered reasonable and necessary for the treatment of the individual's illness or injury only where an expectation exists that the therapy will result in a significant <u>practical</u> improvement in the individual's level of functioning within a reasonable period of time. Where an individual's improvement potential is insignificant in relation to the extent and duration of occupational therapy services required to achieve improvement, such services would not be considered reasonable and necessary and thus are not covered. If a valid expectation of improvement exists at the time the occupational therapy program is instituted, the services would be covered even though the expectation may not be realized. However, in such situations the services would be covered only up to the time at which it would have been reasonable to conclude that the patient is not going to improve. Once a patient has reached the point where no further significant practical improvement can be expected, the skills of an occupational therapist will not be required in the carrying out of any activity and/or exercise program required to maintain function at the level to which it has been restored. Consequently, while the services of an occupational therapist in <u>designing</u> a maintenance program and making infrequent but periodic evaluation of its effectiveness would be covered, carrying out the program is not considered reasonable and necessary for the treatment of illness or injury and such services are not covered.

Generally speaking, occupational therapy is not required to effect improvement or restoration of function where a patient suffers a temporary loss or reduction of function (e.g., temporary weakness which may follow prolonged bedrest following major abdominal surgery) which could reasonably be expected to improve spontaneously as the patient

2-94.8   Rev. 1209 gradually resumes normal activities. Accordingly, occupational therapy furnished in such situations would not be considered reasonable and necessary for the treatment of the individual's illness or injury and the services are not covered.

Occupational therapy may also be required for a patient with a specific diagnosed psychiatric illness. Where such services are required they would be covered, assuming the coverage criteria are met. However, where an individual's motivational needs are not related to a specific diagnosed psychiatric illness, the meeting of such needs does not usually require an individualized therapeutic program. Such needs can be met through general activity programs or the efforts of other professional personnel involved in the care of the patient, because patient motivation is an appropriate and inherent function of all health disciplines which is interwoven with other functions performed by such personnel for the patient. Accordingly, since the special skills of an occupational therapist are not required, an occupational therapy program for individuals who do not have a specific diagnosed psychiatric illness would not be considered reasonable and necessary for the treatment of an illness or injury, and services furnished under such a program are not covered.

Occupational therapy may include vocational and prevocational assessment and training. When services provided by an occupational therapist are related <u>solely</u> to specific employment opportunities, work skills or work settings, they are not reasonable or necessary for the <u>diagnosis or treatment</u> of an illness or injury and are not covered. However, exercise care in applying this exclusion, because the assessment of level of function and the teaching of compensatory techniques to improve the level of function, especially in activities of daily living, are services which occupational therapists provide for both vocational and nonvocational purposes. For example, an assessment of sitting and standing tolerance might be nonvocational for a mother of young children or a retired individual living alone, but would be a vocational test for a sales clerk. Training an amputee in the use of a prosthesis for telephoning is necessary for everyday activities as well as for employment purposes. Major changes in life style may be mandatory for an individual with a substantial disability; the techniques of adjustment cannot be considered exclusively vocational or nonvocational.

Services of support personnel (e.g., occupational therapy assistants) and supplies used in furnishing covered therapy (e.g., looms, ceramic tiles, or leather) are included as part of the covered service. These items and services cannot be billed separately; they must be included in the therapist's bill (see §5252.B).

Rev. 1209   2-94.9

<u>Comprehensive Outpatient Rehabilitation Facility (CORF) Services</u>

2220.   COVERAGE OF PHYSICIANS' SERVICES PROVIDED IN A COMPREHENSIVE OUTPATIENT REHABILITATION FACILITY

A.   Section 933 of P.L. 96-499 (the Omnibus Reconciliation Act of 1980) added to the scope of benefits available to beneficiaries under Part B, rehabilitation services furnished by comprehensive outpatient rehabilitation facilities (CORFs).

Under the amendment, a CORF is recognized as a provider of services, reimbursable on the basis of its reasonable costs. Except for diagnostic and therapeutic services provided by physicians, reimbursement is made by intermediaries acting in the role of Part B carriers (see §§9300 - 9300.2).

B.   Physicians' diagnostic and therapeutic services furnished to an individual patient are not CORF physician's services. If covered, payment for these services is made by the carrier on a reasonable charge basis subject to the same limitations applicable to physicians' services furnished in outpatient hospital settings (see §§A5031 - A5031.3).

When physician's diagnostic and therapeutic services are furnished in a CORF, the claims form must be clearly annotated to show the CORF as the place of treatment.

C.   Certain administrative services provided by the physician associated with the CORF are considered CORF services reimbursable to the CORF by the intermediary. These services include: consultation with and medical supervision of non-physician staff, establishment and review of the plan of treatment, and other medical and facility administration activities.

2-94.10

Rev. 1209

3905.   MEDICAL REVIEW (MR) OF PART B INTERMEDIARY OUTPATIENT SPEECH-LANGUAGE PATHOLOGY (SLP) BILLS

     A.   Claims Documentation.--Medically review each claim referred to Level II or III for outpatient speech-language (SLP) services, regardless of setting. All information must be readable. If possible, use speech-language pathologists to review SLP claims. Obtain the following required information from the provider:

     o   Facility and Patient Identification - (Facility name, provider number, patient name, HICN, age.)

     o   Physician Referral and Date.

     o   Date of Last Certification - Obtain the date on which the plan of treatment for SLP was last certified by the physician.

     o   Diagnosis - The primary medical diagnosis for which services are rendered must be listed first; other diagnoses applicable to the patient or that influence care follow.

     o   Communication Disorder Diagnosis.

     o   Duration - The total length of time services have been rendered (in days) from the date they were initiated for the diagnosis being treated at the billing provider (including the last day in the current billing period).

     o   Number of Visits - The total number of patient visits completed since services were initiated for the communication disorder diagnosis being treated by the billing provider. The total visits to date (including the last visit in the billing period) must be given rather than for each separate billing.

     o   Date of Onset - (Occurrence Code 11) - The date of onset or exacerbation of the communication disorder diagnosis for which services were rendered by the billing provider.

     o   Date Treatment Started - (Occurrence Code 35) - The date services were initiated by the billing provider for the communication disorder diagnosis.

     o   Billing Period - When services began and ended in the billing period (from-through dates).

     o   Medical History - Obtain only the medical history which is pertinent to, or influences, the treatments or tests rendered. Include a brief description of the functional status of the patient prior to the onset of the condition requiring services and any pertinent prior treatment.

     o   Initial Assessment and Date - (At the billing period.)

Rev. 1424   10-75

 o <u>Plan of Treatment and Date Established.</u>

 o <u>Progress Notes</u> - Obtain updated patient status reports concerning the patient's current functional communication abilities/limitations.

 1. <u>Medical History.</u>--If a history of previous SLP treatment is not available, the provider may provide a general summary regarding the patient's past relevent medical history recorded during the initial assessment with the patient/family (if reliable) or through contact with the referring physician. Information regarding prior treatment for the current condition, progress made, and treatment by the referring physician must be provided when available. The level of function prior to the current exacerbation or onset should be described.

The patient's medical history includes the date of onset and/or exacerbation of the illness or injury. If the patient has had prior therapy for the same condition, use that history in conjunction with the patient's current assessment to establish whether additional treatment is reasonable.

The history of treatments from a previous provider is necessary for patients who have transferred to a new provider for additional treatment. For chronic conditions, the history gives the date of the change or deterioration in the patient's condition and a description of the changes that necessitate skilled care.

 2. <u>Assessment.</u>--Approve initial assessment when it is reasonable and necessary for the speech-language pathologist to determine if there is an expectation that either restorative services or establishment of a maintenance program will be appropriate for the patient's condition.

Reassessments are covered if the patient exhibits a demonstrable change in motivation, clearing of confusion, or the remission of some other medical condition which previously contraindicted SLP services. Periodic routine reevaluations (e.g., monthly, bimonthly) for a patient undergoing a SLP program are part of the treatment session and are not covered as separate evaluations. An initial assessment or reassessment that is determined reasonable and necessary based on the patient's condition, may be approved even though the expectations are not realized, or when the assessment determines that skilled services are not needed.

The assessment establishes the baseline data necessary for assessing expected rehabilitation potential, setting realistic goals, and measuring communication status at periodic intervals.

The initial assessment must include objective baseline diagnostic testing (standardized or nonstandardized), interpretation of test results, and clinical findings. If baseline testing cannot be accomplished for any reason, this should be noted in the initial assessment or

10-76

Rev. 1424

progress notes along with the reason(s). The assessment must include a statement of the patient's expected rehabilitation potential.

     3.   <u>Plan of Treatment</u>.--The plan of treatment must contain the following:

        o   Type and nature of care to be provided;
        o   Functional goals and estimated rehabilitation potential;
        o   Treatment objectives;
        o   Frequency of visits; and
        o   Estimated duration of treatment.

     a.   <u>Functional Goals</u>.--Must be written by the speech-language pathologist to reflect the level of communicative independence the patient is <u>expected</u> to achieve outside of the therapeutic environment. The functional goals reflect the final level the patient is expected to achieve, are realistic, and have a positive effect on the quality of the patient's everyday functions.

Assume that certain factors may change or influence the final level of achievement. If this occurs, the speech-language pathologist explains the factors which led to the change of the functional goal. Examples of functional communication goals in achieving optimum communication independence are the ability to:

        o   Communicate basic physical needs and emotional status.

        o   Communicate personal self-care needs.

        o   Engage in social communicative interaction with immediate family or friends.

        o   Carry out communicative interactions in the community.

NOTE: The term "communication" includes speech, language, as well as voice skills.

A functional goal may reflect a small, but meaningful change which enables the patient to function more independently in a reasonable amount of time. For some patients it may be the ability to give a consistent, functional "yes" and "no" response; for others it may be the ability to demonstrate a competency in naming objects using auditory/verbal cues. Others may receptively and expressively use a basic spoken vocabulary and/or short phases; and still others may regain conversational language skills.

     b.   <u>Treatment Objectives</u>--Specific steps designed to reach a functional goal. When the patient achieves these objectives, the functional goal is met.

     c.   <u>Frequency of Visits</u>--An estimate of the frequency of treatment to be rendered (e.g., 3x week).

Rev. 1424   10-77

Length of visits are typically 30, 45, or 60 minutes. Sometimes patients are seen for shorter periods several times a day (for example, three 10 minute sessions or a total of 30 minutes.) Rarely, except during an assessment, are session lengths longer than 60 minutes. If longer times are used, the provider must justify them, by noting that e.g., the patient is exceptionally alert, the number of appropriate activities needing skilled intervention is greater than average, special staff/family training is required. Intensive treatment is sometimes required post-operatively (e.g., tracheoesophageal puncture) or post-onset of disorder (due to intensive family involvement).

       d.   <u>Estimated Duration of Treatment</u>--Identifies the total estimated time over which the services are to be rendered and may be expressed in days, weeks, or months.

       4.   <u>Progress Reports (Treatment Summary for Billing Period)</u>.--Obtain the following:

    o   The initial functional communication status of the patient at this provider setting;

    o   The present functional status of the patient and progress (or lack of progress) specific for this reporting period;

    o   The patient's expected rehabilitation potential; and

    o   Changes in the plan of treatment.

Where a valid expectation of improvement existed at the time services were initiated, or thereafter, the services are covered even though the expectation may not be realized. However, in such instances, approve the services only to the time that no further significant practical improvement can be expected. Progress reports must document a continued expectation that the patient's condition will improve significantly in a reasonable and generally predictable period of time.

"Significant," means a generally measurable and substantial increase in the patient's present level of communication, independence, and competence compared to their levels when treatment was initiated. Do not interpret the term "significant" so stringently that you may deny a claim because of a temporary setback in the patient's progress. For example, a patient may experience a new intervening medical complication or a brief period when lack of progress occurs. The medical reviewer may approve the claim if there is still a reasonable expectation that significant improvement in the patient's <u>overall functional ability</u> will occur. However, the speech-language pathologist and/or physician should document such lack of progress and explain the need for continued intervention.

Documentation includes a short narrative progress report and objective information in a clear, concise manner. This provides you the progress in meeting the plan of treatment, along with any changes in the goals or the treatment plan. Request new plans attached to the original so that you can review the entire plan. However, you must have access to an overall treatment plan with final goals and enough objective information with each claim to determine progress toward meeting the goals.

10-78   Rev. 1424

Consistent reporting is important. For example, if the provider reports that the patient can produce an "m" 25 percent of the time, then reports 40, 60, 90 percent success, you may believe that treatment might be ending. However, if you have the final goal and the objectives, you can see the progress toward that goal and the steps needed to reach it. The speech-language pathologist might state that the final goal is "the ability to converse in a limited environment." One underlying SLP goal might be to "reduce the apraxia sufficiently so the patient can initiate short intelligible phrases with a minimum of errors." Short-term goals may include the patient's ability to initiate easier phonemes before other, more difficult, phonemes. Therefore, the speech-language pathologist has a linguistically and neurologically sound basis for working on one phoneme production before initiating another.

The speech-language pathologist might work on a group of phonemes having a "feature" in common before working on another group. For example, working on all bilabials (since the patient can easily see the movement), might be desirable prior to sounds that are produced more intraorally.

The speech-language pathologist may choose how to demonstrate progress. However, the method chosen, as well as the measures used, generally remain the same for the duration of treatment. The provider must interpret reports of test scores, or comparable measures and their relationship to functional goals, in progress notes or reports. Diagnostic testing should be appropriate to the communication disorder.

While a patient is receiving SLP treatment, the speech-language pathologist reassesses the patient's condition and adjusts the treatment. However, if the method used to document progress is changed, the reasons must be documented, including how the new method relates to the previous method. If the speech-language pathologist reports a subtest score for one month, then a score of a different subtest the next month without demonstrating the subtest's interrelationship, you are not able to judge the progress. Return these claims for an explanation/interpretation. Refer to Level III MR if needed.

     5.   Level of Complexity of Treatment.--Base decisions on the level of complexity of the services rendered by the speech-language pathologist, not what the patient is asked to do. For example, the patient may be asked to repeat a word and the speech-language pathologist analyzes the response and gives the patient feedback that the patient uses to modify the response. The speech-language pathologist may ask staff or family to repeat the activity as a reinforcement. It is the speech-language pathologist's analysis that makes the activity skilled.

     6.   Reporting on New Episode or Condition.--Occasionally, a patient who is receiving or who has previously received SLP services, experiences a secondary or complicating new illness. The provider documents the signficance of any change to the communication capabilities. This may be by pre and post episodic objective documentation, through nursing notes or by physician reports. If the patient is receiving treatment, it might have to be lengthened because of his change in condition. If the patient has completed treatment, a significant change in the communication status must be documented to warrant a new treatment plan.

Rev. 1424   10-79

7.   Qualified Speech-Language Pathologist.--

      o   A person who is licensed, if applicable, by the State in which he/she is practicing, and

      o   Is eligible for a certificate of clinical competence in SLP granted by the American Speech·Language·Hearing Association, or:

      --   Meets the educational requirements for certification, and is in the process of accumulating the supervised experience required for certification.

      o   The speech-language pathologist normally indicates certification status by utilizing CCC-SLP or CFY-SLP:

      --   CCC-SLP - Certificate of Clinical Competence in SLP; or
      --   CFY-SLP - Clinical Fellowship Year in Speech-Language Pathology.

    8.   Certification and Recertification.--SLP services must be certified and recertified by a physician and furnished while under the care of a physician. They must be furnished under a written plan of treatment established by the physician or a qualified speech-language pathologist providing such services. If the plan is established by a speech-language pathologist, it must be reviewed periodically by the physician. The plan of care must be established (reduced to writing by either professional or the provider when it makes a written record of the oral orders) before treatment is begun. When outpatient SLP services are continued under the same plan of treatment for a period of time, the physician must certify at intervals of at least every 30 days that there is a continuing need for them. Obtain the recertification when reviewing the plan of treatment since the same interval of at least 30 days is required for the review of the plans. Recertification must be signed by the physician who reviewed the plan of treatment. Any changes established by the speech-language pathologist must be in writing and signed by the speech-language pathologist or by the attending physician. The physician may change a plan of treatment established by the speech-language pathologist. The speech-language pathologist may not alter a plan of treatment established by a physician.

   B.   Examples of Skilled and Unskilled Procedures.--

   1.   Skilled Procedures.--

      o   Diagnostic and assessment services to ascertain the type, causal factor(s) and severity of speech and language disorders. Reassessment if the patient exhibits a change in functional speech or motivation, clearing of confusion, or remission of some other medical condition which previously contraindicated SLP or audiology services.

o   Design of a treatment program relevant to the patient's disorder(s). Continued assessment of progress during the implementation of the treatment program, including documentation and professional analysis of the patient's status at regular intervals.

o   Establishment of compensatory skills (e.g., air-injection techniques, word finding strategies).

o   Establishment of a hierarchy of speech-language tasks and cueing that directs a patient toward communication goals.

o   Analysis related to actual progress toward goals.

o   Patient and family training to augment restorative treatment or to establish a maintenance program.

2.   Unskilled Procedures.--

o   Nondiagnostic/nontherapeutic routine, repetitive and reinforced procedures (e.g., the practicing of word drills without skilled feedback).

o   Procedures which are repetitive and/or that reinforce <u>previously</u> learned material which the patient or family is instructed to repeat.

o   Procedures which may be effectively carried out with the patient by any nonprofessional (e.g., family member, restorative nursing aide) after instruction and training is completed.

o   Provision of practice for use of augmentative or alternative assessment communication systems.

NOTE: It is only after the patient has established a high level of consistency of performance in a task with the speech-language pathologist, that unskilled techniques can be implemented.

C.   Examples of Statements Supporting and Not Supporting Coverage.--

1.   Statements Supporting Coverage.--Typically, these statements have an objective component which is <u>compared to previous reports</u>, and which demonstrate <u>progress</u> toward a stated functional goal.

EXAMPLES: "Mr. Smith achieved 75 on the Word Subtest on the Johnson Test of Aphasia compared with last month's score of 50 on the same Subtest."

"Mr. Jones achieved a combined score of 352 on the A, B, C, D, and E, subtests this month compared with an overall score of 250 for these same subtests last month."

Rev. 1424   10-81

"Mrs. Jones achieved the next steps in the treatment plan outlined last month (see attached sheet). If she continues at this rate she should complete treatment within the next 2 months."

"Mrs. Jones achieved 75% (7.5 out of 10 or 75 out of 100) on word naming which compares to last month's score of 50% (5.0 out of 10 or 50 out of 100)."

NOTE: Percent should be based on real number count. <u>Interpretation of scores must be presented in progress notes or summary information.</u> The narrative should also contain reference to objective scoring, comparison of previous scores, or treatment plan with present status compared to previous status. This information may be embedded in narrative or attached, however, the reviewer should have access to this information and <u>stated functional goals.</u>

2.   <u>Statements Not Supporting Coverage.</u>--Typically, these statements are subjective, and do not demonstrate progress toward a stated functional goal, or a comparison to previous test scores.

EXAMPLE: "Ms. Jones is very concerned about going home. She has begun smoking again which is causing family as well as physical problems."

"Speech somewhat slurred today."

"Mr. Smith more consistent in responses."

"Mr. Jones has shown significant improvement in his ability to make himself understood."

"Patient is now able to inject air 80% of the time." (No comparison to previous report.)

"Mrs. Smith achieved 75% accuracy on word naming task. (No comparison to previous report)."

"Auditory comprehension improved from moderately impaired to mildly impaired," (by itself, the statement does not offer sufficient objective information.)

D.   <u>Resumption of Treatment.</u>--There are conditions and circumstances that justify resuming treatment after it has been delayed. Obtain verification (when needed for coverage decisions). Examples include:

o   Patient becomes more alert, attentive, cooperative;
o   Patient shows rehabilitation potential;
o   Medical complications cleared;
o   Environmental change improves motivation or communicative capabilities;
o   Progressive nature of disorder warrants further treatment; and
o   Drug or other medical treatment is reduced or ended.

3905.1   <u>MR Considerations</u>.--

   A.   <u>Disorders Typically Not Covered for the Geriatric Patient</u>.--

      o   <u>Stuttering</u> (except neurogenic stuttering caused by brain damage)

          Fluency Disorder
          Cluttering
          Disprosody
          Disfluency

      o   <u>Myofunctional Disorders</u>

          Tongue Thrust

      o   <u>Behavioral/Psychological Speech Delay</u>

   B.   <u>Maintenance</u>.--Approve claims only when the specialized knowledge and judgment of a qualified speech-language pathologist is required to design and establish a maintenance program. By the time the patient's restorative program has been completed, the maintenance program has already been designed, with instructions to patient, supportive personnel, or family. Do not approve a separate charge for establishing the maintenance program immediately after the restorative program has been completed.

Obtain documentation that justifies a provider reestablishing a maintenance program, e.g., loss in previous functional abilities occurs, intervening medical conditions develop, difficulty in communicating with caregivers arises.

The initial assessment should be documented with standardized testing (if possible) to establish base-line data. This is critical if a claim is submitted for care at a future date. Documentation should show that the maintenance program is designed by the speech-language pathologist appropriate to the capacity and tolerance of the patient and the treatment objectives of the physician.

The maintenance program is established when documentation indicates it has been designed for the patient's level of function and instructions to the patient and supportive personnel have been completed for them to safely and effectively carry them out. The documentation must give reasonable assurances that this has occurred. After that point, the services are not reasonable and necessary.

C. Group Treatment.--Generally, group therapy treatment and attendance at social or support groups, such as stroke clubs or lost cord clubs, are not reimbursable. Ensure that the "reasonable and necessary" requirements are met.

D. Total Laryngectomy.--A total laryngectomy is the surgical removal of the larynx. Documentation may involve pre-op/post-op sessions as part of the assessment, to inform the patient, the family, and staff about alternative communication methods, and to provide an immediate means of communication. Documentation includes assessment and any treatment necessary to establish a means of communication using esophageal speech, an artifical larynx (electronic or pneumatic device), a trecheoesophageal puncture prosthesis, and/or other alternate communication methods.

E. Partial Laryngectomy.--A partial laryngectomy is the surgical removal of part of the larynx. Documentation includes the voice problems that require assessment and treatment. Documentation may involve pre-op/post-op sessions as part of the assessment, and to inform the patient, the family, and staff about voice problems. Documentation for rehabilitation also includes the assessment, type of treatment required for the voice disorders, and includes base-line objective data and progress notes.

F. Total Glossectomy.--Total glossectomy is the surgical removal of the tongue. Total glossectomy results in articulation problems that require assessment and may require treatment. Documentation may include pre-op/post-op sessions as part of the assessment, to inform the patient, the family, and staff about articulation disorders, and to provide an immediate means of communication and/or to establish an effective maintenance program. Documentation includes assessment and type of treatment for the articulation disorders. Documentation for articulation treatment involves instruction of compensatory techniques and alternate communication methods if needed.

G. Partial Glossectomy.--Partial glossectomy is the surgical removal of part of the tongue. Documentation should indicate the articulation problems that require assessment and treatment. Documentation may include pre-op/post-op sessions as part of the assessment, to inform the patient, the family, and staff about articulation disorders, and to provide an immediate means of communication following surgery. Documentation includes the assessment and type of treatment for the articulation disorders including base-line objective data and progress notes. Documentation for articulation treatment involves instruction of compensatory techniques and alternate communication methods if needed.

10-84   Rev. 1424

H. Congenital Disorders.--Documentation must always substantiate need, e.g., no previous treatment; the patient's communicative capabilities have recently deteriorated; new, special techniques or instruments have become available; or intervening medical complications have affected SLP communication. Approve claims for maintenance or short-term treatment only if objective documentation supports that need.

I. Alzheimer's Disease.--(Chronic brain syndrome, organic brain syndrome). Objective documentation must indicate the patients' condition, alertness and mental awareness. Documentation must justify that services are needed to establish a reasonable and necessary maintenance program. Review these claims carefully for medical necessity.

J. Chronic Conditions.--Claims for patients with chronic conditions such as MS, ALS, Parkinson's Disease or Myasthenia Gravis can be approved if they document a need for reasonable and necessary short-term care or a need to establish a maintenance program. However, clear documentation must be submitted concerning any prior care or maintenance program designed for the same condition. Approve claims for reasonable and necessary short-term intervention to improve oral and laryngeal strength, speech intelligibility, or vocal intensity, but only when the documentation supports the need to increase function, or to establish a maintenance program.

3905.2   Speech-Language Pathology Terms.--

Agnosia - Inability to attach meaning to sensory information although the physiologic receptor mechanism is intact.

Agrammatism - Impairment of the ability to produce words in their correct sequence; difficulty with grammar and syntax.

Agraphia - Disorder of writing. It may result from a central nervous system lesion or from lack of muscular coordination.

Anomia - Loss of the ability to identify or to recall and recognize names of persons, places or things.

Aphasia - Communication disorder caused by brain damage and characterized by complete or partial impairment of language comprehension, formulation, and use. It excludes disorders associated with primary sensory deficits, general mental deterioration, or psychiatric disorders. Partial impairment is often referred to as dysphasia.

<u>Aphonia</u> - Loss of voice.

<u>Apraxia</u> - (1) Disruption in the ability to transmit a motor response along a specific modality; involves disruption of voluntary or purposeful programming of muscular movememts while involuntary movements remain intact; characterized by difficulty in articulation of speech, formulation of letters in writing, or in movements of gesture and pantomime. (2) In speech, a nonlinguistic sensorimotor disorder of articulation characterized by impaired capacity to program the position of speech musculature and the sequencing of muscle movements (respiratory, laryngeal, and oral) for the volitional production of phonemes.

<u>Dysarthria</u> - Term for a collection of motor speech disorders due to impairment originating in the central or peripheral nervous system. Respiration, articulation, phonation, resonation, and/or prosody may be affected; volitional and automatic actions, such as chewing and swallowing, and movements of the jaw and tongue may also be deviant. It excludes apraxia and functional or central language disorders.

<u>Dysphagia</u> - Difficulty in swallowing. It may include inflammation, compression, paralysis, weakness, or hypertonicity of the esophagus.

<u>Generalization</u> - (1) In conditioning, the eliciting of a conditioned response by stimuli similar to a particular conditioned stimulus. (2) Transfer of learning from one environment to a similar environment; the more similar the environments or situations, the more transfer takes place.

<u>Hard Glottal Attack</u> - Forceful approximation of the vocal folds during the initiation of phonation.

<u>Intonation</u> - Linguistic system within a language which is concerned with pitch, stress, and juncture of the spoken language; a unit with specific communicative import, such as interrogation, exclamation, and assertion.

<u>Lexicon</u> - Total accumulation of linguistic signs, words or morphemes, or both, in a given language; the list of all the words in a language.

<u>Morphology</u> - Component of grammar concerned with the formation of words, the smallest meaningful unit in a language, as a bridge between phonology and syntax.

<u>Obturator</u> - (1) Any structure which occludes an opening. (2) Prosthetic appliance, similar to a dental plate, that forms an artificial palate to cover a cleft palate, designed so that the musculature of the palate and pharynx are able to contract around it.

<u>Paraphasia</u> - Any error of commission modifying a specific word (sound and morpheme substitution) or of word substitution in the spoken or written production of a speaker or writer.

<u>Perseveration</u> - Tendency to continue an activity, motor or mental, once started, and to be unable to modify or stop even though it is acknowledged to have become inappropriate.

<u>Phoneme</u> - Shortest arbitrary unit of sound in a given language that can be recognized as being distinct from other sounds in the language.

<u>Phonological</u> - Component of grammar determining the meaningful combination of sounds.

<u>Pitch</u> - Acuteness or gravity of a tone, dependent upon the frequency of the vibrations producing it and their intensity and overtone structure. The greater the number of vibrations per unit of time, the higher the pitch and the more acute the tone.

<u>Pragmatics</u> - Functional use of language in context. It includes such factors as intention in communication; sensorimotor actions preceding, accompanying, and following the utterance; knowledge shared in the communicative dyad; and the elements in the environment surrounding the message.

<u>Prosody</u> - (1) Physical attributes of speech that signal linguistic qualities such as stress and intonation. It includes the fundamental frequency intensity of the voice, and the duration of the individual speech sounds. (2) Melody of speech determined primarily by modifications of pitch, quality, strength, and duration; perceived primarily as stress and intonational patterns.

<u>Psychoacoustics</u> - Combined disciplines of psychology and acoustics concerned with the study of man's response to sound.

<u>Semantic</u> - Component of grammar concerned with word meanings and meaningful sentences.

<u>Syntactic</u> - Component of grammar concerned with grammatically well formed structures.

3905.3   <u>Acronyms and Abbreviations.</u>--

ADL - Activities of Daily Living.

ALPS - Aphasia Language Performance Scales.

ASHA - American-Speech-Language-Hearing Association.

ASL - American Sign Language.

CVC - Consonant-vowel-consonant.

CPS - Cycles per second. Former unit of measurement for the number of successive compressions and rarefactions of a sound wave within one second of time, now replaced with Hertz (Hz).

Dx - Diagnostic therapy.

MLU - Mean Length of Utterance - Average length of oral expressions as measured by a representative sampling of oral language. It is usually obtained by counting the number of morphemes per utterance and dividing by the number of utterances.

VOT - Voice Onset Time - (1) Time between the release of the stop consonant and the beginning of voicing in the vowel. (2) Time required to initiate sound at the vocal folds.

3905.4   <u>Speech-Language Pathology Tests.</u>--Include but are not limited to:

    A.   <u>Widely Used Adult Language Tests.</u>--

        Ammons Full Range Picture Vocabulary Test
        Aphasia Clinical Battery I
        Aphasia Language Performance Scales (ALPS)
        Appraisal of Language Disturbances (ALD)
        Boston Diagnostic Aphasia Examination (BDAE)
        Communicative Abilities in Daily Living (CADL)
        Examining for Aphasia
        Functional Communication Profile
        International Test for Aphasia
        Language Modalities Test for Aphasia
        Language Proficiency Test (LPT)

Minnesota Test for Differential Diagnosis of Aphasia
Porch Index of Communicative Abilities (PICA)
Revised Token Test
Sklar Aphasia Scale
Token Test for Receptive Disturbances in Aphasia
Hodson Phonological Process Analysis
Clinical Evaluation of Language Functions (CELF)
Western Aphasia Battery

B. <u>Widely Used Adult Articulation Tests</u>.--

Apraxia Battery for Adults (ABA)
Assessment of Intelligibility of Dysarthric Speech
Compton-Hutton Phonological Assessment
Frenchay Dysarthria Test
The Fisher-Logemann Test of Articulation Competence
Iowa Pressure Articulation Test
Templin Darley Test of Articulation

C. <u>Speech and Language Diagnostic Tests</u>.--It is required that an initial assessment (including diagnostic testing, if clinically possible) be performed <u>prior</u> to the commencement of treatment. If you need assistance in understanding tests used, consult your speech-language pathologist consultant or the American·Speech·Language·Association.

Medical Review of Part B Intermediary
Outpatient Physical Therapy Bills

3904.   MEDICAL REVIEW (MR) OF PART B INTERMEDIARY OPT BILLS

    A. General.—The following criteria identify OPT services that your MR staff must review. You may select these cases manually or by computer. You must either select OPT claims for medical review by using the diagnostic edits identified in these instructions or review OPT claims at a 100 percent level. However, if you choose to use any of the diagnostic edits listed in Exhibit I, the visits and/or duration parameters may not be changed without approval from CO. You may review claims in addition to those identified here. If you choose to select claims for review in addition to those identified in Exhibit I, or if you elect to review OPT claims at a 100 percent level, secure approval from your RO and for the criteria you use to select the additional claims. However, you must conform to the MR requirements for all outpatient claims identified in these instructions from rehabilitation agencies, SNFs, hospitals, and HHAs that provide OPT in addition to home health services (bill types, hospital-13, SNF-23, HHA-34, rehabilitation agency, public health agency or clinic-74). These criteria do not apply to inpatient PT services or to PT services provided under a home health plan of treatment or to PT services furnished by CORFs.

The criteria for MR case selection are based on ICD-9-CM diagnoses, elapsed time from start of care (at the billing provider) and number of visits. See Exhibit I for these criteria. Denial of a bill solely on the basis that it exceeds the criteria in these edits is prohibited. The edits are only for selecting bills to review or for paying bills that meet Level I criteria without MR. Also, do not provide automatic coverage, up to these criteria. They neither guarantee minimum coverage nor set maximum coverage limits.

    B. Level I Review Process.—PT edits have been developed for a number of diagnoses. The diagnoses were selected on the basis that, when linked with a recent date of onset, there is a high probability that Medicare patients with those diagnoses will require skilled OPT. The edits do not specify every diagnosis which may require PT, and therefore, the fact that a given diagnosis does not appear in the edits does not create a presumption that OPT services are not necessary or are inappropriate for that diagnosis. Claims may not be approved or denied at Level I for reasons of medical necessity. Claims that pass the edits in Exhibit I and any additional edits approved by your RO may be paid without being subjected to Level II MR.

Evaluate bills at Level I based upon each of the following:

    o Facility and Patient Identification - (facility name, patient name, provider number, HICN, age).

    o Diagnosis - The primary diagnosis for which OPT services were rendered must be listed by ICD-9-CM code first; other Dx(s) applicable to the patient or that influence care must be listed next.

    o Duration - The total length of time OPT services have been rendered (in days) from the date treatment was initiated for the diagnosis being treated at the billing provider (including the last day in the current billing period).

Rev. 1398   10-53

o   <u>Number of Visits</u> – The total number of patient visits completed since OPT services were initiated for the diagnosis being treated by the billing provider. The total visits to date (including the last visit in the billing period) must be given rather than for each separate billing (value code 50).

o   <u>Date of Onset</u> (Occurrence Code 11) – The date of onset of the primary physical therapy diagnosis for which OPT services were being rendered by the billing provider.

o   <u>Date Treatment Started</u> (Occurrence Code 35) – The date OPT services were initiated by the billing provider for the primary physical therapy Dx being treated.

o   <u>Billing Period</u> – When OPT services began and ended in the billing period (from through dates).

C.   <u>Level II Review Process.</u>—If a bill exceeds the limit set in the edits or represents a diagnosis other than one on the edits, refer it to the Level II health professional MR staff. If possible, have physical therapists review OPT bills.

Once the bill is selected for MR, review it in conjunction with medical information submitted by the provider.

1.   <u>Reimbursable PT Services.</u>—Reimburse OPT services only if they meet all requirements established by the Medicare guidelines and regulations. Each bill for OPT services that is subjected to Level II or III MR must be supported with adequate medical documentation for you to make a determination. The documentation must show that the requirements of §§3101.8, 3118.1 and 3148 and in these instructions are met.

2.   <u>MR and Documentation.</u>—When a claim is subsequently referred to Level II MR, use the following pertinent data elements in addition to those used for Level I review:

o   <u>Medical History</u> – Obtain only the medical history which is pertinent to, or influences the OPT treatment rendered, including a brief description of the functional status of the patient prior to the onset of the condition requiring OPT, and any pertinent prior PT treatment.

o   <u>Physician Referral and Date</u> –

o   <u>PT Initial Evaluation and Date</u> –

o   <u>Plan of Treatment and Date Established</u> –

o   <u>Date of Last Certification</u> – Obtain the date on which the plan of treatment was last certified by the physician.

o   <u>Progress Notes</u> – Obtain updated patient status reports concerning the patient's current functional abilities/limitations.

Use the above information along with that in subsection B, to assess the appropriateness of the OPT plan of treatment and the patient's progress relative to diagnosis, date of onset, etc. The medical information supporting a bill must be specific. Documentation written in general terms, e.g, "strength appears to have increased" or "can now reach higher overhead" or "medical history-chronic arthritis" is insufficient. To make an informed MR decision request documentation from the provider when incomplete or inadequate documentation is present. The physician's pertinent evaluations, progress notes and opinions about the patient's need for rehabilitation services, should also be used (when these are available). Obtain this information from the provider regardless of the document type the provider keeps (i.e., it does not matter whether the baseline evaluation is part of the treatment plan, the progress notes or the medical history, obtain and use this information).

3. Medical History.—If a history of previous PT treatment is not available, the provider may provide a general summary regarding the patient's past relevent medical history recorded during the initial evaluation with the patient/family (if reliable) or through contact with the referring physician. Information regarding prior history and treatment by the referring physician must be provided when available.

The patient's medical history, as it relates to the OPT, must include the date of onset and/or exacerbation of the illness or injury. If the patient has had prior OPT for the same condition, use that history in conjunction with the patient's current assessment to establish whether additional treatment is reasonable.

The history of treatments from a previous provider is also necessary for patients who have transferred to a new provider for additional treatment. For example, if surgery has been performed, be aware of the type and date of surgery. The date of onset and type of surgical procedure should be specific for diagnoses such as fractured hip. For other diagnoses, such as arthritis, the date of onset may be general and can be established from the date the patient first required medical treatment. For other types of chronic diagnoses, the history must give the date of the change or deterioration in the patient's condition and a description of the changes that necessitate skilled OPT. For example, a patient that had an amputation several years ago might recently have been fitted with a new prosthesis.

4. Evaluation.—A PT initial evaluation, (excluding routine screening) should be approved when it is reasonable and necessary for the therapist to determine if there is an expectation that either restorative or maintenance services will be appropriate for the patient's condition. Reevaluations should be approved when the patient exhibits a demonstrable change in physical functional ability in order to reestablish appropriate treatment goals, or when required for ongoing assessment of the patient's rehabilitation needs. Initial evaluations or reevaluations that are determined reasonable and necessary based on the patient's condition, may be approved even though the expectations are not realized, or when the evaluation determines that skilled rehabilitation is not needed.

The PT evaluation establishes the baseline data necessary for assessing expected rehabilitation potential, setting realistic goals, and measuring progress. The evaluation of the patient's condition must form the basis for the physical therapy treatment goals.

The evaluation must (when possible) include objective tests and measurements which normally will include functional, strength, and range of motion (ROM) assessments. However, for patients with certain neurological conditions (such as upper motor neuron

Rev. 139 8   10-55 conditions) assessment of strength may not be valid. Where the above tests are not applicable, the physical therapist should document the patient's functional loss and the need for skilled OPT intervention resulting from conditions such as:

     o   <u>Self-Care Dependence</u> - The individual is dependent upon skilled assistance or supervision from another person in self-care activities. These activities include, but are not limited to, signficant functional loss or loss of previous functional gains in the ability to:

       —   Drink;
       —   Feed;
       —   Dress; or
       —   Maintain personal hygiene.

Additionally, this could include care of braces or other adaptive devices.

     o   <u>Mobility Dependence</u> - The individual is dependent upon another person for skilled OPT assistance or supervision in such areas as transfer, gait training, stair climbing, and wheelchair maneuvering activities due to, but not limited to:

       —   Decreased strength;
       —   Marked muscle spasticity;
       —   Moderate to severe pain;
       —   Contractures;
       —   Incoordination;
       —   Perceptual motor loss;
       —   Orthotic need; or
       —   Need for ambulatory or mobility device.

This could involve patients with or without impairment of the lower leg who are partially independent with wheelchair and/or who have significant architectural or environmental barriers.

     o   <u>Safety Dependence/Secondary Complications</u> - A safety problem exists when a patient without skilled assistance cannot handle him/herself in a manner that is physically safe. This may extend to the performance of activities of daily living or to acquired secondary complications which could potentially intensify medical sequelae such as fracture nonunion, or decubiti. Some examples of safety dependence may be demonstrated by high probability of falling, swallowing difficulties, severe pain, loss of skin sensation, progressive joint contracture, and infection requiring skilled PT intervention to protect the patient from further complication.

Each patient's condition calls for assessments which are unique to specific impairments. For example, documentation in the treatment of open wounds or ulcerations require other objective and subjective documentation, such as size and depth of the wound, amount and frequency of drainage, signs of granulation, or evidence of infection, etc.

If the goal for any patient is to increase functional abilities, range of motion, or strength, the initial evaluation must measure (if possible) the patient's starting functional abilities, range of motion and strength. If the assessment indicates that joint range of motion or strength is normal, there should be evidence of this assessment in the initial evaluation or progress notes, e.g., "within normal limits." If objective documentation cannot be accomplished for any reason, this should be noted in the inital evaluation or progress notes along with the reason(s).

   5.   Plan of Treatment.—The PT plan of treatment must include specific functional goals and a reasonable estimate of when they will be reached (e.g., 6 weeks). It is not adequate to estimate "1 to 2 months on an ongoing basis." The plan of treatment must include modalities/procedures, frequency, and duration of treatment. The modalities/procedures must be specific. Changes in the plan of treatment should be submitted with the progress notes.

The plan of treatment must contain the following information concerning the PT treatment:

   o   Type of Modalities/Procedures - Should describe he specific nature of the therapy to be provided. Some examples of PT modalities/procedures are deep heat (e.g., diathermy, ultrasound), superficial heat (e.g., hot packs, whirlpool), and therapeutic exercises and gait training.

   o   Frequency of Visits - An estimate of the frequency of treatment to be rendered (e.g., 3x week).

   o   Estimated Duration - Identifies the length of time over which the services are to be rendered and may be expressed in days, weeks, or months.

   o   Diagnoses - Should include the PT diagnosis if different from the medical diagnosis. For example, the medical diagnosis might be "rheumatoid arthritis." However, the shoulder might be the only area being treated, so the PT diagnosis might be "adhesive capsulitis." In order to establish the PT diagnosis, diagnostic tests must be used whenever possible.

   o   Functional Goals - Should reflect the physical therapist's and/or physician's description of what the patient is expected to achieve as a result of therapy.

   o   Rehabilitation Potential - The therapist's and/or physician's expectation concerning the patient's ability to meet the goals at initiation of treatment.

   6.   Progress Reports (Status Summary(s) Related to the Billing Period).—The physical therapist must provide treatment information regarding the current status of the patient during the course of the billing period. The PT progress notes and any needed reevaluation(s) must update the baseline information provided at the initial evaluation. If there is a change in the plan of treatment, it must be documented in accordance with §3148.3. Additionally, when a patient is continued from one billing period to another, the progress report(s) must reflect comparison between the patient's current functional status and that obtained during the previous billing and/or at the initial evaluation.

Where a valid expectation of improvement exists at the time OPT services are initiated, or thereafter, reasonable and necessary services would be covered even though the expectation may not be realized. However, in such instances, the OPT services are covered only up to the point in time that no further significant functional improvement can be reasonably expected. Progress reports or status summaries by the physician and/or physical therapist must document a continued expectation that the patient's condition will continue to improve significantly in a reasonable and generally predictable period of time. "Significant," in this context, means a generally measurable and substantial increase in the patient's present level of physical functional abilities compared to their level at the time treatment was initiated.

Do not interpret the term "significant" so stringently that you deny a claim simply because of a temporary setback in the patient's progress. For example, a patient may experience a new intervening medical complication or a brief period when lack of progress occurs. The medical reviewer should approve the claim if the services are considered reasonable and necessary and if there is still a reasonable expectation that significant improvement in the patient's <u>overall safety or functional ability</u> will occur. However, the physical therapist and/or physician should document such lack of progress and briefly explain the need for continued skilled PT intervention.

Medical review of rehabilitation claims must be conducted with an understanding that skilled intervention may be needed, and improvement in a patient's condition may occur, even where a patient's full or partial recovery is <u>not</u> possible. For example, a terminally ill patient may begin to exhibit self care, mobility and/or safety dependence requiring PT services. The fact that full or partial recovery is not possible or rehabilitation potential is not present, must not affect MR coverage decisions. The deciding factor is always based on whether the services are considered reasonable, effective, treatment for the patient's condition and they require the skills of a physical therapist, or whether they can be safely and effectively carried out by nonskilled personnel, without physical therapy supervision. The reasons for physical therapy intervention must be clear to you, as well as their goals, prior to a coverage determination. These claims often require review at Level III.

It is essential that the physical therapist document the updated status in a clear, concise, and objective manner. Objective tests and measurements are stressed when these are practical. The physical therapist selects the appropriate method to demonstrate current patient status. However, the method chosen, as well as the measures used, should be consistent during the treatment duration. If the method used to demonstrate progress is changed or comparable measures are used; the reasons for the change should be documented, including how the new method relates to the old. You must have an overview of the purpose of treatment goals in order to compare the patient's current functional status to that in previous reporting periods.

While objective documentation often necessitates range of motion, strength, and other objective measurements; documentation of the patient's current functional status compared to previous reporting period(s) is of paramount importance. The deficits in functional ability should be clear.

Physical therapists must document functional improvements (or lack thereof) as a result of their treatments. Documentation of functional progress must be stated whenever possible in objective, measurable terms. The following illustrates these principles:

o   <u>Pain</u> - Documentation describing the presence or absence of pain and its effect on the patient's functional abilities must be considered in MR decisions. A description of its intensity, type, changing pattern, and location at specific joint ranges of motion will materially aid correct MR decisions. Documentation should describe the limitations placed upon the patient's self care, mobility and/or safety, as well as the subjective progress made in the reduction of pain through treatment.

Transcutaneous electrical nerve stimulation (TENS) uses surface electrodes and electrical current to interrupt pain pathways and sensation of pain through peripheral nerves. Generally, it is covered on a trial basis for up to 1 month. Any trial period extending beyond 1 month must be documented as to reason and medical necessity. Approve such claims only when the documentation supports the need to assess the patient's suitability for continued treatment with TENS. When it is determined that TENS should be continued as therapy and the patient has been trained to use the stimulator, it is expected that the stimulator will be employed by the patient at home. Payment may be made under the prosthetic devices benefit for the TENS stimulator. Payment may not be approved for continued OPT treatments with TENS. (See Coverage Issues Manual 35-46 and 65-8.)

o   <u>Therapeutic Exercise</u> - The objective documentation should support the skilled nature of the exercise program, and/or the need for design and establishment of a maintenance exercise program. The goals should be to increase functional abilities in self care, mobility or patient safety. Documentation should indicate the goals and type of exercise provided and the major muscle groups treated.

Approve claims when the therapeutic exercise, because of documented medical complications, the condition of the patient, or complexity of the exercise employed, must be rendered by, or under, the supervision of a physical therapist. For example, while passive and active assistive exercise may often be performed safely and effectively by nonskilled personnel, the presence of fracture nonunion, severe joint pain, or other medical or safety complications may warrant skilled PT intervention to render the service and/or to establish a safe maintenance program. In these cases, the complications and the skilled services they require, must be documented by physician orders and/or physical therapy notes. To make correct MR decisions, the patient's losses and/or dependencies in self care, mobility and safety must also be documented. The possibility of adverse effects from the improper performance of an otherwise unskilled service does not make it a skilled service unless there is documentation to support why skilled PT is needed for the patient's medical condition and/or safety.

Approve establishment and design of a maintenance exercise program to fit the patient's level of ADL, function, and any instructions supportive personnel and/or family members need to safely and effectively carry out the program. Reevaluation may be approved when reasonable and necessary to readjust the maintenance program to meet the changing needs of the patient. There must be adequate justification for readjusting a maintenance program, e.g., loss of previous functional gain.

o   <u>Cardiac Rehabilitation Exercise</u> - Physical therapy is not covered when furnished in connection with cardiac rehabilitation exercise program services (see Coverage Issues Manual 35-25) unless there also is a diagnosed noncardiac condition requiring it e.g., where a patient who is recuperating from an acute phase of heart disease may have had a stroke which requires PT. (While the cardiac rehabilitation exercise program may be considered by some a form of PT, it is a specialized program conducted and/or supervised by specially trained personnel whose services are performed under the direct supervision of a physician.) Restrictions on coverage of PT do not affect rules regarding coverage or noncoverage of such services when furnished in a hospital inpatient or outpatient setting.

o   Gait Training - The documentation must support that the skilled gait training is designed to restore functional abilities (or to design and establish a safe maintenance program) which can reasonably be expected to improve the patient's ability to walk or walk more safely. Documentation should clarify the patient's gait deviation, current functional abilities and limitations, and/or safety dependence during gait. Documentation should identify the gait problem being treated, e.g., to correct a balance/incoordination and safety problem or a specific gait deviation, such as a Trendelenberg gait. The type of gait deviation requiring skilled intervention, the functional limitations in mobility, the patient's understanding or lack of understanding of the gait training, and the amount of assistance needed during training is needed to make correct review decisions. The documentation must differentiate skilled gait training rendered from assistive walking, when the patient is walking repetitiously and merely improving distance or endurance (assistive or nonassistive).

o   Transfer Training - The documentation should describe the patient's functional limitations in transfer ability that warrant skilled PT intervention. Documentation should include, the special transfer training needed and rendered, and any training needed by supportive personnel and/or family members to safely and effectively carry it out. Transfer training should be approved when the documentation supports a skilled need for evaluation, design and effective monitoring and instruction of the special transfer technique for safety and completion of the task.

Documentation that supports only repetitious carrying out of the transfer method, once established, and monitored for safety and completion of the task is noncovered care.

o   Electrical Nerve Stimulation - Approve reasonable and necessary electrical stimulation to delay or prevent disuse atrophy, but only where the documentation indicates that the nerve supply (including brain, spinal cord and peripheral nerves) to the muscle is intact, and other nonneurological reasons for disuse are causing atrophy. (See Coverage Issues Manual §35-77.)

Electrotherapy for the treatment of facial nerve paralysis, e.g., Bell's palsy is not a covered service. (See Coverage Issues Manual §35-72.)

Approve functional electrical stimulation (FES) used to test the suitability for improving the patient's functional ability when documented in the PT notes as lost. For example, to stimulate the dorsiflexors of the ankle, thereby, reducing toe drag during the swing-through phase of gait.

o   <u>Biofeedback Therapy</u> - Approve claims when the documentation indicates that it is reasonable and necessary for the patient for muscle reeducation of specific muscle groups, or for treating pathological muscle abnormalities of spasticity, incapacitating muscle spasm, or weakness.

Deny claims where the documentation supports treatment for ordinary muscle tension states or for psychosomatic conditions. (See Coverage Issues Manual 35-27.)

o   <u>Fabrication of Temporary Prostheses, Braces, and Splints</u> - Approve reasonable and necessary fabrication of temporary prostheses, braces and splints, and any reasonable and necessary skilled training needed in their safe and effective use. The documentation must indicate the need for the device and training.

D.   <u>Certification and Recertification.</u>—To meet Medicare guidelines, PT services must be certified and recertified by a physician. They must be furnished while the patient is under the care of a physician. The OPT services may be furnished under a written plan of treatment established by the physician or a qualified physical therapist providing them; however, if the plan is established by a physicial therapist, it must be reviewed periodically by the physician. The plan of care must be established (reduced to writing by either professional or the provider when it makes a written record of the oral orders) before treatment is begun. When OPT services are continued under the same plan of treatment for a period of time, the physician must certify at least every 30 days that there is a continuing need for them. Obtain the recertification at the time the plan of treatment is reviewed since the same 30 day interval is required for the plan's review. Any changes to the treatment plan established by a physicial therapist must be in writing and signed by the physicial therapist or by the attending physician. Recertifications must be signed by the physician who reviewed the plan of treatment. The physician may change a plan of treatment established by the physical therapist, the physical therapist may not alter a plan of treatment established by a physician.

E.   <u>Physical Therapy Forms.</u>—Documentation may be submitted on a specific form or may be copies of the provider's record. You may require a specific form if you find it more efficient than using provider records; however, it must capture the MR information required by these instructions. If you choose to require one, show the OMB clearance number. The information must be complete. If it is not, request the missing information and return the bill for the additional information. The information you require to review the bill is that required by a physical therapist to properly treat a patient.

F.   <u>Post-Pay Sample.</u>—Review a random sample (percent determined by HCFA) of the bills that pass all edits (i.e., are paid without MR), using either a random number generator or terminal HICN. Each quarter, assign a new random number generator/HICN. This is unnecessary if you medically review all OPT claims.

Conduct a post-pay MR on each claim selected in accordance with subsection C. Determine a provider's denial rate by combining the prepay and postpay denials for the same quarter. Calculate the rate by dividing the provider's total charges that you have determined noncovered by the total charges submitted by the provider in that quarter. Place providers having a 5 percent or higher denial rate in any quarter on 100 percent prepay MR in the subsequent quarter. Providers with a denial rate of less than 5 percent for two (2) consecutive quarters may be removed from 100 percent MR. Handle new providers according to your existing procedures.

Consider investigating abnormal trends uncovered during the post-pay sample review by conducting special Level I edit studies. Alert your RO to your findings, along with recommendations, prior to taking any corrective action or procedural changes.

G. Completion of the MR Report.—

1. Report of OPT MR Activities.—Complete and submit within 15 calendar days of the close of the calendar quarter, the following report (Exhibit II).

Submit reports to:

> Health Care Financing Administration
> Office of Program Operations Procedures, BPO
> 1-H-3 Meadows East Bldg.
> 6325 Security Blvd.
> Baltimore, MD 21207

Send a copy to the regional administrator.

2. Completing the OPT Edits Report (Exhibit II).—

NOTE: If you perform 100 percent MR, see subpart 3 below.

Item 1 - Intermediary Number - Enter your assigned identification number.

Item 2 - Intermediary Name - Enter your corporate name.

Item 3 - Intermediary Contact - Enter the name of the individual responsible for completing the report.

Item 4 - Telephone Number - Enter the phone number of the individual named in Item 3.

Item 5 - Reporting Quarter - Enter the last month of the reporting quarter and the year (i.e., December, March, June, or September).

Item 6 - Date of Completion - Enter the date the report is forwarded to HCFA.

Item 7 - Total Bills to Pass Edits - Enter the total number of OPT bills (revenue code 42x) that were paid or identified for payment without MR. (Bills passing edits.)

Item 8 - Charges for Bills Passing Edits - Enter the dollar amount (charges) for OPT bills passing edits.

Item 9 - Total Number of Bills Suspended - Enter the number of bills suspended for MR as a result of your edits.

Item 10 - Charges for Bills Suspended - Enter the dollar amount (charges) for bills suspended for MR.

Item 11 - Total Number Bills Paid - Enter the number of bills paid as billed after MR.

Item 12 - Total Number of Bills Denied - Enter the number of bills denied (including partial denials) after MR.

Item 13 - Charges Denied - Enter the dollar amount (charges) denied after MR.

Item 14 - Review - Based upon HCFA's, RO's, or your edits, or 100 percent review. Enter the applicable category.

        3.   Co.npleting the OPT Edits Report (Exhibit II) With 100 Percent Medical Review.—

Item 1 through Item 6 - See subpart 2.

Item 7 - Total Number Bills to Pass Edits - Enter 0.

Item 8 - Charges for Bills Passing Edits - Enter 0.

Item 9 - Total Number Bills Suspended - Enter the number of OPT bills reviewed.

Item 10 - Charges for Bills Suspended - Enter the sum of all OPT charges for all bills reviewed.

Item 11 - Total Number Bills Paid - Enter all OPT bills which were subjected to MR and subsequently paid.

Item 12 - Total Number of Bills Denied - Enter the number of OPT bills denied (including partial denials) after MR.

Item 13 - Charges Denied - Enter the dollar amount (charges) denied after MR.

Item 14 - Review - Based upon HCFA's, RO's, or your edits, or 100 percent review. Enter the applicable category.

NOTE: If you peform 100 percent review, skip the following items.

        4.   Co.npleting of Items 15-18 of the OPT Screens Report (Exhibit II).—

Item 15 - Number Sample Bills Reviewed - Enter the number of OPT bills selected for sample review from the bills passing the edits.

Item 16 - Charges for Sample Bills Reviewed - Enter the dollar amount (sum of the charges) on the OPT bills selected.

Item 17 - Number Sample Bills Denied - Enter the number of OPT bills denied after MR.

Item 18 - Charges for Sample Bills Denied - Enter the dollar amount (sum of the charges) denied following MR.

Rev.   1398

EXHIBIT I
OUTPATIENT PHYSICAL THERAPY EDITS

The following edits are not based on normative treatment. It is prohibited to deny a bill solely on the basis that it exceeds the edits. The edits are for selecting bills for Level II MR.

Edit Identification Number	Diagnosis	ICD-9-CM	Number of Visits	Duration (MO.)
1.	CA (category A)	162.0-163.9	7	1
	CA (category B)	165.0-165.9	24	2
		170.0-172.9		
		174.0-174.9		
		191.0-192.9		
		195.3-195.8		
		201.0-201.9		
		225.0-225.9		
		238.0-238.1		
		239.6		
2.	Parkinson's Disease	332.0-332.1	13	1
3.	Meningitis/Encephalitis	320.0-323.9	16	2
	Intracranial and intraspinal abcess	324.0-324.9		
	Huntington's Chorea and other choreas	333.4-333.7		
	Spinocerebellar disease	334.0-334.9		
	ALS and other motor neuron diseases	335.2-335.9		
	Other diseases of the spinal cord	336.0-336.9		
	Multiple Sclerosis	340		
	Demyelinating Diseases of CNS	341.8-341.9		
	Hemiplegia (old)	342.0-342.9		
	Paralytic syndrome	344.0-344.9		
	Late effects of CVA	438		
4.	Cerebral hemorrhage, occlusion, stenosis	430-434.9	32	3
	CVA, acute	436		
	Concussion, Loss of consciousness without return to previous level	850.4		
	Intracranial injury including those with skull Fx	800.7-800.8		
		801.7-801.8		
		803.2-803.3		
		803.7-803.8		
		804.7-804.8		

10-64

Exhibit 1 (Cont.)

Edit Identification Number	Diagnosis	ICD-9-CM	Number of Visits	Duration (MO.)
5.	T.I.A.	435.0	7	1
	Other ill defined cerebrovascular diseases	437.0-437.9		
	Late effects of viral encephalitis	139.0		
6.	Other paralytic syndromes, paraplegia quadriplegia	344.0-344.9	39	3
	FX of vertebral column with spinal cord injury	806.0-806.5 806.8-806.9		
	Spinal cord injury	952.0-952.9		
7.	Post-herpetic polyneuropathy	053.13	19	2
	Neurosyphilis	094.0-094.9		
	Late effects polio	138		
	Diabetes with neurological manifest	250.6		
	Bell's palsy	351.0		
	Disorders of peripheral nerves	353.0-359.9		
	Other peripheral nerve injuries	953.0-957.9		
8.	Diabetes with peripheral circulatory disorders	250.7	13	1
	Diseases of circulatory system	402.0-429.9		
	Raynaud's/Buerger's/PVD	443.0-443.9		
	Thrombophlebitis lower extremity	451.0-451.2		
	Lymphedema	457.0-457.9		
9.	Hansen's Disease	030.0-030.9	29	2
	Gas gangrene	040.0		
	Diabetes with ulcer manifestation	250.8		
	Varicose vein with ulcer	454.0-454.2		
	Cellulitis	681.0-682.9		

Rev. 1398   10-65

Exhibit 1 (Cont.)

Edit Identification Number	Diagnosis	ICD-9-CM	Number of Visits	Duration (MO.)
	Other local infection of skin	686.0-686.9		
	Chronic ulcer of skin	707.0-707.9		
	Gangrene	785.4		
	Open wounds	875.0-884.2 890.0-894.2		
	Burns (second degree)	941.2 942.2 943.2 944.2 945.2 946.2 949.2		
	Post traumatic wound infection	958.3		
	Infection of stump	997.62		
10.	Tuberculosis respiratory	010.0-012.8	7	1
	Acute Bronchitis	466.0-466.1		
	Bronchopneumonia	480.0-486		
	Bronchitis, emphysema	491.0-492.8		
	Asthma, unspecified	493.9		
	Bronchiectasis	494		
	Chronic airway obstruction	496		
11.	Diffuse disease of connective tissue	710.0-710.9	18	2
	Arthropathy associated with infection	711.0-711.9		
	Arthropathy associated with other disorders	713.0-713.8		
	Rheumatoid arthritis and inflamatory polyarthropathies	714.0-714.9		
	Gouty arthopathy	274.0		
12.	Osteoarthrosis and allied disorders	715.0-716.9	13	1
13.	T.M.J. disorders	524.6	13	1
	Internal derangement of joint, other derangement of joint and other unspecified disorders of joint	717.0-719.9		

10-66   Rev. 1398

Exhibit 1 (Cont.)

Edit Identification Number	Diagnosis	ICD-9-CM	Number of Visits	Duration (MO.)
14.	Dorsopathies Osteoporosis Pathological Fx Aquired spondylolisthesis Anomalies of spine	720.0-724.9 733.0 733.1 738.4-738.5 756.10-756.12	13	1
15.	Peripheral enthesopathies and allied syndromes disorders of muscles, tendons and their attachments and other soft tissues	725-729.9 (excluding 727.1 and 727.4)	13	1
16.	Gait disturbances due to weakness, incoordination debility and/or after surgery or Fx	780.7 739.6 731.2 799.3 V66.4	13	1
17.	Fx of vertebral column without cord injury Late effects of Fx spine	805.0-805.9 905.1	14	1
18.	Fx of pelvis Fx of femur	808.0-808.9 820.0-821.39	18	2
19.	Fx of patella Fx of tibia and fibula Fx of ankle, tarsals, metatarsals	822.0-822.1 823.0-823.9 824.0-825.39 827.0-827.1	18	2
20.	Fx of humerus Fx of radius and ulna Fx of carpals Fx of metacarpals and phalanges Fx of radius and ulna	811.0-819.1	18	2

Exhibit 1 (Cont.)

Edit Identification Number	Diagnosis	ICD-9-CM	Number of Visits	Duration (MO.)
21.	Dislocations	830.0-339.9	18	2
	Crushing injury	927.0-929.9		
22.	Sprains and strains	840.0-848.9	13	1
	Late effects of strains, sprains, dislocations	905.6-905.7		
	Contusions	922.0-924.9		
	Injury, other unspecified	959.1-959.9		
23.	Amputation	885.0-887.7	32	3
		896.0-897.7		
24.	Burns (3rd and 4th degree)	941.3-941.5	32	3
		942.3-942.5		
		943.3-943.5		
		944.3-944.5		
		945.3-945.5		
		946.3-946.5		
		949.3-949.5		
25.	Joint replacement	V43.6	19	2
26.	Fitting and adjustment of prosthetic care	V52.0-52.1	13	1
	Removal internal fixation device	V54.0		
	Orthopedic aftercare	V54.8-V54.9		
	Late effects FX	905.1-905.5		
	Late effects tendon injury	905.8		
	Late effects amputation	905.9		

10-68

Rev. 139 8

Exhibit IV

Report of Outpatient Physical Therapy Bills

FI # (1) _____   FI Contact (3) _____   Reporting Qtr (5) _____

FI name (2) _____   Telephone No (4) _____   Date of Completion (6) _____

For all bills processed, fill in Items 7-13.

7 Total # Bills to Pass Screens	8 Charges for Bills Passing Screens	9 Total # Bills Suspended	10 Charges for Bills Suspended	11 Total # Bills Paid	12 Total # Bills Denied	13 Charges Denied

14.   Review based on: _____

For sample (of bills passing screens) review, fill in Items 15-18.

15 #Sample Bills Reviewed	16 Charges for Sample Bills Reviewed	17 #Sample Bills Denied	18 Charges for Sample Bills Denied

Rev. 1398   10-69

☆ U.S. GOVERNMENT PRINTING OFFICE: 1988 - 2 0 1 -8 1 8 /8 0 3 1 2